Satir Family Camp

*An Intentional Community Living
Virginia Satir's Legacy*

by

D1601690

Elsa Ten Broeck
Mary D. Garrison

Science and Behavior Books, Inc.
Palo Alto, California

Printed in the United States of America

Library of Congress Control Number 2008930465

ISBN 978-0-8314-0094-1

Editing by Rain Blockley
Printing by BookMasters, Inc.

Contents

Acknowledgments

The authors wish to thank the Satir Family Camp and all of the members who contributed to this book. Without their honesty and cooperation, we could not have written this book. We also extend a special thanks to those who read our manuscript to provide input and feedback that helped shape the final product. Their insight was invaluable. Finally, we extend a special appreciation to Linda Leviton for her illustrations and to Becky and Bob Spitzer and the staff of Science and Behavior Books, Inc. for their support of our work.

Foreword

by Russell Haber, Ph.D., ABPP
SFC Facilitator (1994–present)

Years before I joined the therapeutic team at Satir Family Camp, my wife and I participated in a month-long Satir Process Community in 1979. After just five days of small-group exercises, romantic relationships flourished in this group of sixty family therapists, even though most were married. The scene of newly formed couples reminded me of transitory summer-camp romances. Satir's skillful approach of fostering self-esteem, safety, congruence, and personal growth resulted in the group becoming intimate, figuratively and literally.

I found the experience to be an odd paradox. Here we were learning about creating change in families from Virginia Satir, the "Mother of Family Therapy," and at the same time, many participants were putting the integrity of their own families at risk. When I asked Virginia about that phenomenon, she told me that she was very concerned about the other, non-attending family members. She always held them in her field of vision and tried to help workshop participants plan for how to re-enter their families. Nevertheless, some families were unable to incorporate the transformation of one of its members.

I believe Virginia created Satir Family Camp to provide a place where therapists could bring their families with them and learn experientially about how families can optimally live, work, heal, and grow together. I know that Virginia, who birthed many communities, was particularly proud of her experimental community of therapists and their families exploring, growing, and being together in a family camp.

This intentional growth community, which now serves all sorts of family and individual units, often feels to me like Camelot. A community in a beautiful natural setting dedicated to supporting each person's quest "to become more fully human." A place where you learn about families through the experience of living in a community of families. A place that respects everyone's voice deeply, from those of the toddlers through those of the octogenarians.

Two of my favorite times of the day happen at the camp's fire pit. In the morning, a group of campers wakes up together by drinking cappuccino around a fire. In the evening, the many generations of camp members play games, share stories, and make music around a blazing fire. Also, many extemporaneous moments are very special. For instance, I was walking across a field to find two younger boys in a squabble. As I was about to intervene, one of the teens ran over and helped the two boys find a better way to resolve their differences. On the same walk, a five-year-old girl gave me a flower. At that moment, it dawned on me that SFC is a place where everyone takes responsibility for the community's welfare.

In my role as camp therapist, I have found SFC to be a community dedicated to the welfare of its members and the larger community. The therapy sessions help build a culture that embraces support for those curious about learning new ways of handling repetitive problems. The sessions also provide a context for being known in the camp, learning new ways to cope with problems, and receiving support from fellow campers. Different campers chose the venue that works best for them. For instance, some men save most of their deepest sharing for the men's group because that is the place in the community where they feel the most safe.

The facilitators meet every night and process what is happening in the various groups. Often, intersecting issues are occurring in the entire camp, specific subgroups and families, the governing council, and in the community facilitator system. It is a good thing that we have a fun and close-knit system of facilitators, because we spend so much time together.

I write, too, with deep appreciation for my cuddle group of fellow facilitators: Laura Dodson, Maureen Graves, Tom Graves, Shirley Kirby, Malcolm Anderson, Rhea Merck, and especially my wife, Karen Cooper-Haber. Also, my son's (Nathan Haber) passionate commitment to SFC brought more of our family into camp and more of camp into our family.

In addition to the magical moments in the community, a lot of hard work occurs. This entails balancing the needs, propensities, personalities, and structure in this willful community of approximately 125 campers. I learned so much about SFC from reading this delightful book. The book deftly balances the many stories that have shaped SFC with a clear description of the dynamics of community formation. Having read this book, I now know why I get nervous on Thursdays, why safety is so important, why a Pulse Committee exists to control rumors, why people had such investment in the governing committee not losing control of the camp to the facilitators, and even why concern was so high about spraying insecticide to control the plentiful mosquitoes. The history of seminal stories illuminates the present functioning of the camp. As poignantly quoted in the book by one of the current SFC board members (p. 158):

> What makes us succeed as a community is that we look at our dark side and shine a light on it. We also work very hard to deal with our dark side. We keep learning and each time we go through a struggle on a community level we get stronger as individuals and as a community.

This book illuminates both the shadows and rays of sunlight of the camp. Most of all, it captures the magic that Virginia Satir dreamed about prior to 1978. For me, SFC manifests the best parts of Virginia's work: a community devoted to learning to live with creativity, high self-esteem, centeredness, respect, and congruence. Her methods—including Temperature Reading, family therapy, Parts Parties, Family Reconstruction and her recommended twelve hugs per day for growth—work well to achieve her goal of a community that supports the integrity of the family and each individual in "becoming more fully human."

Satir Family Camp has indeed been a successful experiment. It is a story that is worth being told. Thank you, Elsa Ten Broeck and Mary Garrison, for bringing the magic of SFC into print.

Part One

Introduction

In 1977, Virginia Satir created a community known as Satir Family Camp, which brought families to live together in the wilderness for one week each year. That community continues to this day, as both a living legacy to Virginia and one of her best-kept secrets. This book is the first written account of Satir Family Camp (SFC) and the therapeutic work Virginia did there. It shares the camp's history and describes how the community has grown and changed over the years. Using stories, illustrations, and photographs, the book demonstrates how SFC utilizes Virginia's theories, techniques, and teachings to support and guide a unique communal experience now being shared by a third generation of Satir Family Campers.

We use two voices to depict SFC. In one voice, we describe the history and tell the stories; in another, we analyze the different stages of intentional community development. This book shows how a community of families can live together and practice Virginia's principles for "becoming fully human." It also discusses some of the significant challenges the community has faced over the past quarter-century. Growing beyond Virginia's initial dream, the camp has not only survived for over twenty-five years but has thrived even in the most difficult of times. We include an analysis of how Virginia both created some of those challenges and provided the knowledge and skills to deal with them.

Throughout this retrospective, readers find stories and statements that reflect the experiences of Satir Family Camp members as well as friends and colleagues from Virginia's life. In some places, we have quoted people directly; in others, we describe events that happened at camp. To assure confidentiality, we have changed the names of campers who participated in those events. To help illustrate how the sfc community developed, we have also created certain stories. The characters in those stories are composites rather than actual campers.

In all instances, actual or fictional, we have tried to be faithful to the voices of the people who are or who have been part of the community.

Finally, readers can discover how Virginia's life, principles, and models influenced and shaped the wonderful mystery of this intentional community. After careful study of her work and discussions with her colleagues, we also postulate a model of community development that we believe Virginia might have envisioned.

1

Definition

On a warm morning one early April, Nelson, his wife Phyllis, and their daughter Mia, age 7, packed up their Ford station wagon and began a twenty-five-year journey that would change their lives fundamentally as individuals and as a family. On that first trip, Nelson remembers thinking: "What am I doing here? I've never camped in my life, and now I'm going to into the wilderness for a week with a bunch of people I don't know! I bet they've been camping all their lives."

As they turned off California's scenic Coast Highway and began climbing into the hills that surround Big Sur, Nelson's concerns spiraled into panic. To calm himself, he reviewed their gear: tent, chairs, utensils, groceries, suitcases, and duffel bags full of clothes, blankets, and toys. "I wonder if I'm going to have to carry all this stuff to my campsite?" he muttered as he pulled into the grassy meadow that he assumed was the entrance to Satir Family Camp.

All around him, Nelson heard people greeting each other. Some called out to Phyllis, who went rushing off to return greetings with hugs and exclamations. "Man," thought Nelson, "I'm not going to make it through this week if these people are going to be doing this hug thing all the time."

As Phyllis chatted with two women she had met at a Virginia Satir conference, Nelson looked around. A few men were involved in greetings, but most seemed intent on organizing their gear in front of their cars. Nelson followed suit and soon realized a significant difference between his family's stuff and that of their fellow campers. In front of most cars were carefully packed tents, camping gear, and perhaps one duffel bag per person. In front of his station wagon lay his tent, stuffed back into its box as well as he could manage (after his trial attempt to put the tent up in the back yard). Around the tent, spread out in ever increasing circles, were Mia's toys, Phyllis's suitcases, Nelson's suitcases, boxes of food and "special supplies."

Dressed in a bright shirt, shorts, and sandals, a slim man carrying a clipboard came by to introduce himself as Felix, part of the Welcoming Group. As he offered to help Nelson get "a little more organized," it dawned on Nelson that he was not at the camp but at an arrival point. He saw that people around him were climbing onto a flatbed truck. Felix quietly explained that everything had to be trucked into camp, and space on the truck was a bit limited. Without sarcasm, he suggested that perhaps Nelson and Phyllis could re-evaluate their gear and decide what was critical and what could be left behind.

Having rejoined them, Phyllis gave Felix her 100-watt smile and said, "Sure, no problem," while Nelson thought, "Sure, if we have all week to reorganize." Surprisingly, with some help from another family, they had just met, Nelson and Phyllis quickly divided their things into a small "essential" pile and a much larger "non-essential" pile. Suddenly, it was their turn to climb onto the truck.

After surviving their arrival blunders, Phyllis and Nelson began to relax and look around. Chattering people were filling the truck's benches. Some appeared to be old friends; others, acquaintances; and some seemed to know only their immediate families. Felix climbed aboard and made introductions, including that of Harry, the driver. At first, Nelson tried to remember each name. He quickly lost interest in other campers, however, when Felix suggested that people hang on to the truck with one hand and their kids with the other. Felix banged the side of the truck and hollered, "Let's go!" and they rumbled off. Phyllis held onto Mia, Nelson put one arm around Phyllis and grabbed firmly to the side of the truck with his other hand.

After the road's first descent, when the gears shifted abruptly and the whole group tumbled toward the front of the truck, Nelson once again thought, "What am I doing here?" Nevertheless, he helped Phyllis and Mia rearrange themselves, shared some laughter with the family who helped him repack, and looked around at the majesty of his surroundings. Each bend took the group farther away from their cars, their belongings, and their daily lives, and deeper into the wonder and peace of the earth. Trees soared and the heat of the day lifted. As Nelson took in Mia's look of amazement and Phyllis's air of relaxation, he thought, "Okay, I can probably do this for a few days."

Following a half-hour trip of grinding gears, laughing people, and shouting children, the truck stopped. Nelson realized that here, at last, was Satir Family Camp. The center of activity was a flat area filled with broad tree stumps and surrounded by a grove of towering redwood trees. Flowing through the middle of the clearing was a creek, which was the focus of the children's interest. A primitive kitchen was set up near the creek. Mesh bags holding other families' dishes hung from several ropes strung between trees close to the clearing.

Earlier arrivals mingled with the latest group, some running to help unload the truck while others clustered in small groups in intense discussion. Nelson climbed down from the truck, relieved to be on firm ground, and looked up at the massive redwoods. He wondered, "Now what?"

Suddenly standing before him was a tall woman with curly, sandy blond hair. She wore glasses and was dressed in a blue windbreaker, white blouse, and a khaki skirt. When she reached out to take Nelson's hand in both of hers and hold his gaze with her intense blue eyes, Nelson felt as though this woman had known him all his life. Quietly, she said, "Welcome to Family Camp, I'm Virginia Satir. Can I give you a hug?"

Virginia the Person (1916–88)

In the same way that she affected Nelson on his first day there, Virginia had a larger-than-life presence at SFC. To understand SFC completely—its development as well as its current organization—it is first necessary to understand Virginia and the forces that influenced her life. Virginia (née Pagenkopf) Satir was born on June 26, 1918. She lived with her mother, father, and four siblings on a family farm in Wisconsin. Both her parents were children of German immigrants who came to the United States in the late 1800s. As a child, Virginia experienced significant economic poverty and emotional deprivation. Her father was an alcoholic and, for most of Virginia's childhood, her mother was emotionally unavailable. Several times during her childhood and adolescence, Virginia went to live with members of her extended family because her parents were either too ill or too poor to care for her.

Her paternal grandparents lived with Virginia's family when she was very young. "Old man Pagenkopf had begun to slip into some kind of psychosis and . . . engaged in a scene that so frightened little Ginny [Virginia] that she dreamt about it for the next forty years or so"

(Brothers, 1998, p. 16). Later in her life, Virginia learned that this "scene" was her grandfather, during a psychotic episode, chasing his wife around the table with a butcher knife while Virginia's mother was nursing newborn twins and trying to keep two-year-old Virginia safe (*ibid*, pp. 10–11).

Virginia's life was affected not only by her parents' and grandparents' emotional struggles but also by her mother's religious beliefs. Mrs. Pagenkopf was a devout Christian Scientist who chose religious intervention over traditional medicine. These convictions had serious physical repercussions during Virginia's early childhood. When she was about two years of age, she lost her hearing as the result of an untreated ear infection. Four years later, her hearing returned spontaneously, but this significant if temporary deafness had already affected her early development markedly (Spitzer, 2006).

Meanwhile, at age 5, Virginia suffered a ruptured appendix. It was only her father's decision to intervene and take her to the hospital that prevented her death. In this instance, Virginia was hospitalized for over two months while recuperating from the operation (Suarez, 1998). Although Virginia later discussed these events as simply among many difficult events in early childhood, it is not difficult to imagine how they must have traumatized her as a young child.

Her mother's ability to cope as a wife and mother was greatly strained by the birth of medically fragile twins only eighteen months after the birth of her first child. Virginia relates that after the twins were born, her mother pushed her away. "Very early there was the feeling that my mother hated me and that my father was weak and ineffectual and I was supposed to be Queen Mary—to carry the honor of the family somehow" (in Brothers, 1998, p. 17).

These early life experiences started Virginia on a lifetime quest to understand families and their impact on an individual's development. In all her work, she identified early childhood experiences as having the greatest influence on how people function as adults. Certainly, her own family experiences bear this out. Virginia struggled throughout her life with the impact of her conflicted and nonnurturing family environment. Although she was known for her extraordinary professional warmth and charisma, she was both removed and remote in her personal relationships. As a young adult, she married twice: first to Gordon Rogers, a soldier she met at a train station while he was on leave from service in World War II; and then to Norman Satir. Although she became an expert in family issues and family therapy, her own two marriages ended in divorce.

Fritz Perls, both a professional colleague and close friend, described Virginia as a "gypsy." He further described her personal connections: "You have projected your need for an understanding family, and, correspondingly, are family-phobic yourself. Your dreams to settle down remain dreams" (in Brothers, 1998, p. 9).

Those who worked closely with her were particularly aware of the contrast between Virginia the professional and Virginia the private woman. Barbara Jo Brothers, a long-time colleague, described these contradictions in her introductory chapter of the sensitive biography *Virginia Satir: Her Life and Circle of Influence* (1998, p. 48):

> Those who worked closely with her in later years experienced this paradoxical reticence alongside her great warmth and sensitivity to others. . . . Genius therapist though she was, and in direct contrast to what she taught, Virginia never learned how to get enough emotional support from others. She almost always kept to herself that which was most important to her.

An interchange Brothers had with Virginia clearly demonstrates this contradiction. Virginia began the interchange by saying, "Do you know that I love you? I helped birth you, you know," referring to an earlier therapeutic training session. Brothers reached out to Virginia (Brothers, 1998, p. 21):

> Flooded with the memory and the intensity of her suddenly bringing the reality into my awareness, I couldn't think of anything appropriate to say that would acknowledge the depth of my appreciation in that moment. I did want her to know yes, I know that you love me. I turned and hugged her.

Describing Virginia's reactions to the physical contact, Brothers states, "I wondered at how wooden she felt in response" and then described her own confusion about "that subtle distancing quality in an otherwise extraordinarily warm and nurturing woman" (Brothers, 1998, p. 22).

Virginia herself described the conflict she felt about physical intimacy during a training on Family Reconstruction; "I couldn't stand for people to touch me for years" (Brothers, 1998, p. 22). This statement was made by a woman well known for advocating that everyone have at least six hugs a day to survive emotionally.

At sfc, Virginia both worked as the facilitator/therapist and created an environment where, as a "family-phobic" woman, she could have an intense but time-limited family experience. A long-time camper and colleague described Virginia's relationship with SFC:

> Virginia did not have much of a personal or family life. She had limited contact with her birth family or her adult daughters. Avanta and Family Camp were her family. As a result, SFC has been influenced not only by Virginia the professional, but also by Virginia the person, with all her needs. Virginia was a dichotomy between professional commitment and consistency, and personal hypocrisy. She was a brilliant woman who was always professional when "on," but when she was "off" and relating to people on a personal level, she was easily triggered by such little things. And when she was triggered, she was quick to go into blame. She could be a dictator and authoritarian in the way she worked with people in the organizations. She just wanted things to go as she wanted, and expected everyone to do as she said. She was a real micromanager. At the same time, Virginia never used her extraordinary power for self-aggrandizement. She never viewed Family Camp as "hers." In fact, Virginia always wanted camp to evolve into a community that did not depend upon a single leader.

Virginia the Professional (1949–78)

Virginia's work and various influences on her professional life also illuminate events that led to and shaped SFC. Her extraordinary intelligence helped her escape the conflicted legacy of her childhood. It also helped her develop the skills required to excel in her professional life. She taught herself to read by age 3, entered high school at 12, and enrolled in college by 16 (Brothers, 1998, p. 25).

She began her professional life as a teacher but soon moved on to study social work, later explaining that (Brothers, 1983, pp. 48–49):

> I was always looking for information for how things could be better for people. I wanted to understand what was going on. I never went into social work to become "a social worker." I went into social work to find information to help me understand people.

In 1948, Virginia received her Master's degree in social welfare from the University of Chicago School of Social Service Administration. After graduation, she worked full time at the Chicago Home for Girls, where she became involved with two sisters, Mary and Ruth. As she did throughout her life, Virginia combined her professional and personal life by offering her home to Mary and Ruth. They were emancipating and had no family to help in their transition from adolescence to adulthood (Brothers, 1998, pp. 40–42).

Between 1943 and 1950, Virginia married her first husband, suffered a life-threatening ectopic pregnancy (which left her unable to have children of her own), parented Mary and Ruth, and moved from Chicago to Texas. Gordon Rogers served in the military during much of their marriage (Brothers, 1998, pp. 40–42). When the family lived in Texas, Virginia worked at the Child Guidance Clinic in Dallas. In early 1950, after her marriage began to fail, Virginia and the two girls returned to Chicago. Shortly after, Mary and Ruth emancipated from Virginia's care and returned to their hometown. Virginia, depressed and overwhelmed by the impact of all the changes she had faced, realized that she needed to address her increasing depression. She entered analysis, which she described in an interview in 1974 (in Brothers, 1998, pp. 45, 49):

> It limited [the way I could act] tremendously. I am certain that experience, which came at a time when I was really hurting, set new boundaries. But they were negative boundaries. . . . When I was through with it [analysis], I said to myself, "There's gotta be more than this" because, actually, I see the whole thing of psychoanalysis as a rather pessimistic thing about the hopefulness in people.

Through her work with families, she developed a model for treatment that focuses on each person's strengths and avoids labeling anyone's behaviors. In this model, the client is an equal partner in the treatment process rather than the recipient of it (Brothers, 1998, pp. 45, 49). Virginia's unique approach to the treatment relationship was a forerunner of today's client-centered philosophy found in medicine, mental health, and social services.

Her willingness to experiment with different approaches to therapy led to her first family therapy session. A mother of a young woman she was seeing in therapy phoned Virginia to complain about her daughter's treatment (Brothers, 1998, p. 52). Virginia felt she could learn more about the mother's concern as well as her client if she met jointly with them both. She invited the mother to attend her daughter's next session. After the first joint session's success, Virginia realized there were other family members who could provide even more information. She invited the client's father and siblings to attend the following session. The success of these sessions led to the creation of what she called *conjoint family therapy* (Brothers, 1998, p. 50).

Virginia initiated this treatment when it was considered unprofessional even to have two different clients sitting in the waiting room at the same time. Throughout her life and career, however, she went against prevailing wisdom when an action made sense and was helpful to the client.

By 1955, Virginia had provided family therapy to over 400 families. She discovered that when she worked with all members of a family at the same time, she could observe how communication and interactions among family members affected each member as individuals as well as the family as a whole (Brothers, 1998, pp. 51–52).

She first reported on her innovative work at local professional meetings in Illinois (Brothers, 1998, p. 53). It was not until she moved to California in 1958, however, that her work became both recognized and appreciated by the mental health profession. By the 1960s, it was clear that Virginia would devote her life to the mission of helping others achieve their full human potential (Brothers, 1998, p. 2): "All my work and writings are toward this one aim: becoming more fully human. . . . I make no apologies for moving in totally different ways and I hope to move those ways on a mass level."

Virginia began her career in California as a co-founder of the Mental Research Institute (MRI) in Palo Alto, along with Dr. Don Jackson and Dr. Jules Riskin (Brothers, 1998, p. 56). They established MRI, in Virginia's words, "to look at the relationship between the health and illness of individuals and its relationship to the total family interaction" (in Brothers, 1998, p. 60). They also established the institute to conduct scientific research on families. The research focus required therapists to do intensive work with a very limited number of families.

Virginia, always a hands-on learner, found this approach limiting. She was anxious to work with many people and to inform others about what she was learning. Her preferences led her to concentrate on training and educating mental health professionals. At MRI, she worked directly with families while also teaching and lecturing about her observations and understanding of family systems. During this time, she published her seminal work, *Conjoint Family Therapy* (1964). As she lectured widely on conjoint family therapy, communication, self-esteem, and her unique treatment methods, her reputation grew.

The 1960s and 70s were a fertile time for persons like Virginia who were committed to enhancing human growth and development. Virginia was naturally drawn to the activities at Esalen, a conference and retreat center located in Big Sur, California. As described on their website:

> Esalen was founded in 1962 as an institute based on an abiding belief in the untapped potential of all people to learn, to love, to feel deeply, and to create. The Institute's purpose is to seek knowledge through the integration of seeming opposites—mind and body, East and West, action and meditation, the US and the USSR.

From 1965 to 1968, Virginia was in residence at Esalen as director of training. Her experiences there affected her work with families, as she described: "I got into what we call the affective domain; I was bringing another whole growth dimension into my work. That was the beginning of a lot of new things" (in Brothers, 1998, p. 64). The Esalen years also brought about lifetime changes for herself. Sheila Wild, an early Satir Family Camper, remembers Virginia describing her first visit to the famous hot tubs at Esalen:

> Virginia told us how she got into her bathing suit and walked down to the hot tub, only to realize that everyone in the tub was nude. So, typical Virginia, she just shed the bathing suit and joined right in. Virginia never had any problems moving into new environments and taking on new ideas.

Barbara Jo Brothers (1998, pp. 66–67) described how these new ideas changed the way Virginia worked with families between 1965 and 1968.

> In the 1965 [session], she had worn a beige suit as she conducted the interview; everybody sat in chairs; and all her interventions were verbal. In 1968, she was wearing a bright-colored long dress. She engaged the family—who were part of the audience except for their time on stage—in sculpting, demonstrations using ropes, and a variety of other forms. The difference was more than merely obvious; it was striking.

In many ways, Esalen became the model for much of Virginia's future work. Located in an isolated area on the coast of California, surrounded by hot springs and waterfalls, Esalen let participants leave behind the mundane world and enter a magical place that helped center them and explore their humanness. Esalen participants discovered new and uncharted areas of human relationships, spirituality, and science. Virginia's years at Esalen were filled with new learning, including those listed on its website:

> Many new practices, new ways of thinking and being, have been either created or brought to wider public attention by Esalen. These include Gestalt Training, Rolfing, Esalen Massage, Psychosynthesis, Open Encounter, Interracial Encounter, Somatics, Confluent Education, and Integral Transformative Practice.

For several years, Virginia participated actively in these programs. Among others, she worked directly with Fritz Perls, leader of the Gestalt therapy movement;, Eric Berne, leader of Transactional Analysis; and Ida Rolf, creator of the Rolfing technique. Through her Esalen experiences, she learned the importance and power of teaching about not only information but also the feelings and emotions related to that information (Brothers, 1998, p. 64). Esalen also gave her the concept of residential trainings in remote settings that teach and challenge not only people's intellects but their emotions.

Following her work at Esalen, Virginia began to offer mental health practitioners her own unique training seminars. Brothers described how Virginia viewed her evolving work style (1998, pp. 67–68):

> Since 1968, she had learned much more about systems, the integration of right- and left-brain learning and "about how we take in things." In places where she had previously relied on intuition, she now had cognitive handles. She was free to make clear and more open use of the information. . . . Virginia told me that she knew she "developed everything intuitively" and that her "right brain is always ahead of her left brain."

By the early 1970s, Virginia had established herself as a leading mental health educator and clinician. She ended her formal relationships with both MRI and Esalen and began working with people throughout the world. As early as 1961, she presented at the first meeting of the International Association of Social Psychiatry. For the ensuing twenty-seven years, she trained mental health professionals in Germany, Israel, England, Canada, France, Scandinavia, China, Hong Kong, eastern Europe, Venezuela, and Central America. Her final international trips were to Central America and the then Soviet Union (Brothers, 1998, pp. 71, 73). Her worldwide influence can be gauged by the extraordinary number of Satir Institutes throughout the world (Avanta Network, 2007).

As a therapist and trainer, Virginia established a number of events and organizations to provide and teach family therapy. She organized wilderness camps that provided therapy for families and training for therapists in intensive one- or two-week camping trips. In 1969, she conducted her first month-long residential training session for therapists in the United States (Brothers, 1998, p. 76). By 1981, these residential trainings evolved into month-long "Process Communities" that she offered on an annual basis right up to the time of her death.

Meanwhile, in 1977, Virginia founded the Avanta Network as the vehicle for organizing and delivering her trainings. This organization was her primary business endeavor, received her personal as well as professional bequests, and continues to the present. Avanta was and continues to be staffed by Virginia's closest friends as well as business partners. As its website explains (Avanta Network, 2007):

> Her vision was to help empower people to reach their full potential. Virginia invited those who had trained with her and shared her vision to join Avanta. Since its early years, then, Avanta has been a forum for developing ideas, techniques, skills and training. Since Satir's death in 1988, Avanta has carried on her work through national and international conferences, workshops and training efforts, as well as through the efforts of individual members.

In 1970, Virginia held a meeting of what she called "One Hundred Beautiful People." She brought the group together, she said there, to foster connections among people she knew and felt could benefit from meeting each other. Virginia was obviously the common denominator among those in attendance. From that meeting, the group organized the International Human Learning Resources Network (IHLRN). Some still call it the Hundred Beautiful People. Today, both it and Avanta continue the work Virginia began over fifty years ago.

Virginia's international work is carried on at the Institute for International Connections for Personal and Cultural Growth (ICC), founded in 1990. According to its website, the ICC:

> promotes cross-cultural understanding and collaboration in developing peace-oriented, democratic systems. . . . Inspired by the pioneering family systems therapist, Virginia Satir, ICC uses a multi-layered approach to change, involving the individual, family, community and workplace.

Satir Change Theory and Change Model

Over her professional lifetime, Virginia developed many theories about individuals and family systems. Understanding how consistent and universal change exists in all of life, she developed a Theory of Change and a Change Model to teach her unique views. Rather than help people learn to cope with change, she encouraged people to accept and embrace change as the vehicle that helps us live a full life. Virginia described *change* as "an internal shift that in turn brings about external change" (Satir et al.,1991, p. 85). She defined *conscious change* as "the effort to develop a different sense of being, different expectations and perceptions, a different way of handling feelings and more functional ways of coping" (*ibid*, p. 93).

Virginia did not see change as extinguishing or eliminating problems. Rather, she saw it as an action that helps individuals "transform" what already exists into something new (Satir, Banmen, Gerber & Gomori, 1991, p. 87). For Virginia, one achieves greater freedom of choice and greater responsibility for one's inner process as well as for one's behavior through the change process (*ibid*, p. 92).

Although she viewed change as natural and constant, Virginia understood that the way individuals experience or react to change varies. Many individuals and families function at a survival level and do not believe change is possible. They remain in a status quo that is often painful but provides a false sense of safety by virtue of its familiarity. Motivation to move from this state may come from internal pain, an external expression of symptoms relating to that pain, or an external threat, such as legal action. Virginia was convinced that (Satir et al., 1991, pp. 86–88):

> Change . . . especially internal change . . . is possible for everyone regardless of age or other circumstances. Each individual contains all the knowledge that he or she needs within him- or herself. It is the individual, however, not a therapist or other person outside the individual, who must ultimately decide whether to change.

To move from survival mode to high self-esteem and congruence, a person or family must make the conscious decision to change. Making a willing change requires being in touch with one's life force, taking whatever risks are necessary, and being willing to acquire new awareness at a cognitive, emotional, and visionary intentional level. This happens at the six stages of change that make up the Satir Change Model, described in the ensuing sections.

Stage One: Status Quo

Individuals and families generally live, or seek to live, in a state of balance. A troubled individual or unhealthy family system lacks that balance because the individual's needs are unmet or individual family members must contribute more than they receive from the family system. This unbalance can result in people feeling anger, fear, disappointment, lack of closeness, and limited intimacy. These feelings may eventually result in problems for the individual or family system. Change generally occurs for the individual or system when a significant event forces the individual or system to confront the issues that create the imbalance (Satir et al., 1991, p. 100).

Stage Two: Foreign Element

The stage called Foreign Element begins with the introduction of an unfamiliar factor, usually from outside the individual or system (Satir et al., 1991, p. 100). This often occurs because the individual or one member of the system articulates the need for change to someone outside the system (Satir et al., 1991, p. 98).

Stage Three: Chaos

The third stage, Chaos, usually occurs when the individual looks at him- or herself or the system looks at itself. By recognizing, acknowledging, and examining routine expectations and reactive patterns, the individual or system initiates change (Satir et al., 1991, p. 107). Moving from status quo to new behavior almost always requires a period of chaos because the system is operating in ways that are no longer based on old rules and therefore predictable (*ibid,* p.108). During this phase, anxiety is high. "Any new way is unintegrated while the old is no longer fitting, so there is distress and continued imbalance" (Schwab, 1990, p. 110). This is also the phase when healing begins. While in the Chaos stage, individuals consider new perceptions of self and others and can rearrange, restructure, update, and change their perceptions and expectations (Satir et al., 1991, p. 110).

Stage Four: New Options and Integration

When the individual or system changes perceptions and expectations, the New Options and Integration stage begins. Individuals and families now use dormant resources, integrating various personality parts and re-evaluating past and present expectations. Persons and systems in this stage let go of many survival patterns of coping and accept new ways of being.

In this stage, people learn to differentiate between body clues that go with old experiences and those that accompany new leanings (Satir et al., 1991, p. 114).

Stage Five: Implementation

Moving to new options can be challenging because past patterns are automatic, reactive, and comfortable. The Implementation stage involves practicing many new behaviors, ways of relating, looking and seeing, connecting and relating with others, enjoying intimacy, and validating self and others (Satir et al., 1991, p. 115). Because making these changes is hard work, individuals and families usually need ongoing support during this stage to practice and integrate behavior. Similar to the Integration phase, Implementation occurs over time, generally in ongoing therapy.

Stage Six: New Status Quo

In the New Status Quo stage, individuals and systems have achieved a healthier equilibrium and relate more fully and on a more functional level than before their change. A new sense of comfort replaces the familiarity of old behaviors or systems. A new set of predictions develops about how the system operates, and revised self-images and new hopes emerge. Greater spontaneity and creativity are set free, and an enhanced sense of well being occurs (Satir et al., 1991, p. 118).

The process of change continues throughout life. Even when a new status quo exists, change will inevitably occur again. As long as life continues, new circumstances arise that challenge the status quo. Individuals and systems that have made changes in the past often become more comfortable with the process and can accept and often welcome both the challenges and the change process as part of "reaching a more fully functioning way of being"(Satir et al., 1991, p. 124).

The Satir Change Model describes energy that is applied to homeostasis in the self, in couple relationships, and in families. The energy found in each stage of the Change Model helps move the homeostasis toward growth and development. At a community level, the energies of individuals merge to create an entirely new dynamic and identity, sometimes called the *Gestalt*. In the same way that change creates energy that affects the homeostasis of individuals, change on a community level creates energy that affects the homeostasis of the community and drives its development.

The Intentional Community Development Model

This book uses the Satir Change Model to discuss how individuals and families function within the community. We then expand on that model and use our own Intentional Community Development Model to analyze and understand how intentional communities develop and change. The accompanying table indicates the relationship between the two models.

Throughout their development and existence, communities cycle through the five stages of the Intentional Community Development Model. The following sections describe each stage in more detail.

**Relationship of the Intentional Community Development Model
to the Satir Change Model**

Stages of Community Development	Energy Functions of the Satir Change Model Stages
1. **Definition**: community defines its rules of operation	*Status Quo*: energy to maintain the balance of the existing structure
2. **Establishment**: community creates a structure to meet the basic needs of its members	*Status Quo*: energy to maintain the balance of the existing structure
3. **Rebellion**: community identifies the unmet needs of members of the community and demands modifications to the structure	*Foreign Element*: energy focuses on identifying unmet needs *Chaos:* energy focuses on unbalancing the system
4. **Redefinition**: community amends its structure to more effectively address the needs of the community at higher levels than basic survival	*Integration*: energy focuses on analysis of patterns and defining new terms and conditions
5. **Synergy**: community utilizes the new structure to achieve greater goals	*Implementation*: energy focuses on utilizing the new structure and finding a comfortable new balance
6. **Ennui**: community enjoys success and begins to identify new challenges and philosophize about future	*New Status Quo*: abundant energy is diversified to allow individuals more time for questioning and debating the existing structure

Stage 1: Definition

In the initial stage of Definition, members of the community define the purpose of coming together and their goals for working and living in the community. They also define the roles and rules of leadership, basic survival, communication, solving problems, and making decisions.

During this stage, the structure of the community is just emerging and little opposition tends to emerge within the group. This initial cooperation generally stems from the members' desire to establish the community as well as respect for the community's creators. The energy at work is that of the Status Quo stage of the Change Model, in which system members collaborate to establish balance by maintaining the current situation. At this stage, members defer to leaders who present ideas and have the energy to advocate for their implementation.

Stage 2: Establishment

In the Establishment stage, people implement the roles and rules developed during the Definition stage, and the community enjoys an initial semblance of continuity and stability. A key factor contributing to the stability is the community's ability to meet members' basic needs. In the Establishment stage, members also feel secure because they understand their place and their role in the community. This is a time of tentative comfort, which corresponds to the energy of the Status Quo stage in the Satir Change Model. This energy continues to focus on creating a balance that allows members of the community to work together and make the adjustments necessary for the community to function. This does not necessarily suggest that people' have their needs met equally or that the community always functions in a healthy manner. Rather, it simply means that the community functions without overt conflict in this stage.

Stage 3: Rebellion

In the Rebellion stage, community members identify and express dissatisfaction with the community, and they demand change. Community energy now shifts from working together to maintain the balance to focusing on unmet needs of members. The shift usually occurs when one or more community members feel that the existing balance is not meeting the needs of all members equitably.

Usually, internal dissatisfaction or the introduction of new members constitute the Foreign Element that creates this shift. New members often question the status quo of an established community. They question community definitions, roles, communication, resource disbursement, and accepted methods for making decisions and solving problems. Other members then question those same written and unwritten elements.

Fueled by the energy of Chaos, the third stage of the Satir Change Model, community members rebel against the rules of community processes. With these challenges to the status quo, new and unpredictable patterns can emerge. As the structure that has previously served the community comes under scrutiny, a series of trial-and-error attempts to redefine and restructure the community also occurs.

Stage 4: Redefinition

In the fourth stage, Redefinition, the community evaluates various attempts to redefine and restructure during the Rebellion Stage. It looks at these proposals in light of the community's original purpose and goal, agreed on in the Definition stage. If the members decide to change the original goal, the community returns to the Definition stage and develops new premises and definitions. If the community continues under its original stated purpose, the Redefinition stage proceeds, propelled by energy of the Integration stage of the Satir Change Model.

This energy fuels an examination of changes identified in the Rebellion stage as well as the rapid integration of the new ideas, resources, and expectations. The community may choose to redefine some parts of itself, such as the roles, leadership, communication, and problem-solving or decision-making structures.

Once the community accepts these changes, group pressure rapidly arises to re-establish a new sense of balance. This pressure can create a climate in which members conform to the majority or the loudest opinion simply because of the anxiety and unpredictable nature of the Rebellion stage. The community wants to return to the comfort and balance that existed in the earlier stages.

Stage 5: Synergy

In Synergy, the community fully implements new definitions and changes that emerged in the Redefinition stage. During this fifth stage of intentional community development, group members use the new definitions and accept the redefined structure. Integrating the new ideas, resources, and expectations is fueled by energy of the Satir Change Model's fifth stage, Implementation.

New growth becomes possible because the community has returned to homeostasis. People can now focus on how to utilize the new structure to the community's best advantage. In the Synergy stage, a community can concentrate a tremendous amount of power on considering and achieving higher goals. This is because all of the separate pieces of the community's structure are functioning as an organized system.

Synergy is the stage in which communities achieve their greatest success. Communities that reach the Synergy stage are able to focus on activities such as membership drives, building expansion, or financial campaigns. However, as Virginia Satir postulated in her Change Model, change is inevitable and a necessary part of growth and development. As such, the stage of Synergy is never everlasting and frequently leads to the sixth and final stage.

Stage 6: Ennui

In the Ennui stage, the community utilizes the energy of the Change Model's final stage, New Status Quo. More energy is now available within the community because it functions as a whole, pooling everyone's power to create reserves from which the community may draw. Individuals also use this energy for specific interests and endeavors. In Ennui, community members function at a level that is more self-aware and personally responsible. The community structure is working well in this stage, and both the community and individual members are successful. Individuals can focus on personal growth, development, and prosperity.

Due to the very essence of this stage—individual exploration and the lack of challenges for the community as a whole—individual members often eventually suggest, demand, or otherwise orchestrate opportunities to debate the existing status quo. This debate often throws the community back into Rebellion to work through the stages again, albeit with different tools and resources now in place.

The Cycle of Intentional Community Development

The accompanying flow chart shows how community development starts, stops, and cycles back into itself along a natural and expected continuum. Development moves back and forth according to the energy available to propel progress: sometimes moving forward steadily, sometimes regressing to earlier stages. No stage has a defined time limit. In Redefinition, the cycle can either move forward to Synergy or cycle back within itself to the beginning stage, Definition. When a community cycles back to Definition, the development cycle begins again.

Cycle of Community Development

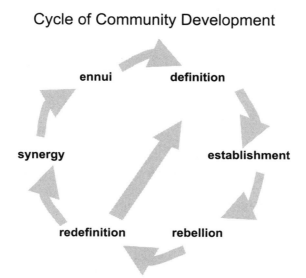

Congruence

The concept of congruence explains how Virginia's techniques help a community move through the challenges of each developmental stage. Most of the techniques and tools described in this book are used to help individuals and communities achieve *congruence*, "a state of being and a way of communicating with ourselves and others" (Satir et al., 1991, p. 65). Virginia considered a fully functional human being to have achieved congruence (Satir et al., 1991, p. 65). She described three levels of congruence, as follows.

Level 1. Feelings

Congruent individuals are aware of their feelings and can acknowledge and accept them without denial or projection. Individuals can manage their feelings in a wholesome way and enjoy the positive feelings that are part of being human (Satir et al., 1991, p. 68).

Level 2. The Self

Congruent individuals have achieved a state of wholeness and inner centeredness that lets them manifest high self-esteem and join in harmony with others. "They are at peace with themselves, with others, and in relation to their context" (Satir et al., 1991, p. 68).

Level 3. Life Force

Congruence is reflected through an awareness of the interconnectedness among individuals, communities, and "a universal life force that creates, supports, and promotes growth in human and other natural forms" (Satir et al., 1991, pp. 68–69). Virginia further described this level of congruence (p. 81):

> When I can be in touch with another person's spiritual energy, and him or her with mine, there is a change in the state of consciousness. We each have the whole world within us, and we each have special functions. We are not attached to one another but connected by the spaces between us. We are part of the one universal whole. I am part of the whole and also the whole.

When individuals are congruent, they have awareness and acceptance of self, others, and the context in which they live. Congruence is particularly important when individuals join together to create an intentional community. Congruent communication helps to identify and state the definitions that underlie the community's purpose (Satir et al., 1991, pp. 69–73). Congruence helps create effective leaders who can guide the community through the Definition stage and into the Establishment stage. Congruence helps communities deal with Rebellion and provides the skills needed to move the community from Rebellion into Synergy. Finally, congruence provides communities with the skills needed both to recognize and deal with the changes encountered in the stage of Ennui.

Virginia designed her personal and professional interests to help her achieve congruence and live a congruent lifestyle. The Satir Family Camp let her engage in some of her favorite pursuits, including family design work, building relationships, networking, mentoring and modeling for developing therapists, and exploring planned communities. At sfc, she focused her work at a community level, despite having no blueprint for doing intensive family work in large groups or for intentional community development. The community allowed her to explore new interventions and methods of fostering individual, family, and community growth.

In compiling the history of sfc, it became clear that every aspect of Virginia's life and work there has contributed to the intentional community it is today. As in all historic analysis, it is much easier to understand how different events have shaped development by looking at those events over time. Not all of Virginia's ideas, interventions, and boundaries were positive. It appears that at times she had a master plan in mind; at other times, it seems that the community has developed in reaction to and almost in spite of Virginia.

2

Establishment: How It All Began

In 1972, Jackie Schwartz, a mental health therapist, attended a Virginia Satir wilderness camp in the high Sierras. Along with eight other therapists, she joined Virginia on a two-week encampment designed to train therapists by providing intensive family therapy to seven families. Along with one other supervising therapist, Virginia supervised seven family therapists who worked with the individual families. The entire group hiked into a camping area at Dardanelles Lake, California. Support staff packed in supplies and created a makeshift kitchen to provide all the meals. In the true sense of a wilderness camp, each family and therapist slept in a tent and worked together even when it rained. One therapist worked with one family on a daily basis. Virginia supervised the therapists and worked with the community as a whole. As Schwartz said (2006):

> It was such an intense and wonderful experience. When it was over, I knew I wanted to share that experience with my family and decided right then and there to organize a similar camp for mental health therapists and their families. And that was how Family Camp got started. The specifics came together during one of Virginia's Hundred Beautiful People meetings. The only time I could get Virginia to meet with me was at 7 a.m. in the hot tub. So Michele and Bud Baldwin, Virginia, and I sat together and talked about how to offer a family camp for mental health therapists. We just designed the program right there in the hot tub!

Ms. Schwartz sent announcements of the first camp to people who had attended Virginia's trainings, and word of mouth circulated among people Virginia knew. To assure that therapists could commit to attend the entire event, the first camp was a one-week event. The original program melded the wilderness camps design with trainings for mental health professionals. Jackie Schwartz (2006) recalled:

> I got a lot of responses from therapists who were either single or in a couple relationship. Despite the pressure I got from these people to attend as well as the pressure I felt financially when we did not get a lot of family enrollment, I held firm to the idea that this was a Family Camp. I wanted at least two thirds of the attendees to be families. It was really touch and go whether we would get enough people to enroll but the last family signed up the week before camp and it happened.

In 1977, ninety-five people—ranging in age from under eight months to eighty years and coming from as far as Israel and Canada—attended the first camp. Several multigenerational families participated. The camp was held at the Presbyterian Conference Grounds in Pacific Palisades, a semi-rural area just outside of Los Angeles, California. The campgrounds provided more luxuries than the original wilderness camps. Each family had a cabin, and the entire group had easy access to the Los Angeles metropolitan area.

Many of the families had teenage children who quickly developed a group identity. They chose to bunk together in a dormitory, and a therapist whose work focused on adolescents helped them organize a teen group to address their issues separately from their parents and other adults.

The adults created a women's group and a men's group. These self-selected groups met following the evening session. Neither group had a leader or a particular agenda. As Schwartz (2006) explained, "There was just so much positive energy generated from the sessions with Virginia that people wanted to keep talking and sharing ideas."

Virginia offered three daily training sessions in which she discussed and demonstrated family therapy concepts. All members of the family attended these trainings.

> Virginia worked very hard to make the sessions interesting to the kids as well as the adults. She was a natural ham and the kids just loved her. She would involve them in some of her demonstrations and she always used examples that the kids could identify with. Virginia made all the decisions about how to handle her sessions and in particular who would do work. Most people came to camp wanting Virginia to do therapeutic work with their families. They made that

known to Virginia but she made the final choice of the families. I know she made sure that in addition to helping the particular family she worked with, she chose families that would allow her to provide the whole group with information and strategies they could use in their own therapeutic practice. [Schwartz, 2006]

The formal camp program also included Temperature Reading each morning (described fully in Chapter 8) so the whole group could discuss issues and concerns. Temperature Reading was often the occasion when Virginia identified people who would work with her that day. She also held "family conclaves" in the evenings. The conclaves consisted of two to four families and a therapist assigned to work with the small group.

Various camp activities occurred during the week. People chose to participate or not based on their individual interests. Wednesday was a free day. The first year, Jackie organized a tour of unusual places in Los Angeles. Eight people began the tour at 3:30 a.m. with a visit to the flower mart and then the produce market, a meal at The Pantry (a unique Los Angeles restaurant), and such sites as the Bradbury Building and the Grand Central Market. The group was back at camp by 11:30 a.m. and had the rest of the day to catch up on sleep. Others used the free day to swim in the pool at the campgrounds, go to Disneyland, or simply decompress from the intensity of the week's work. The camp also hired a camp masseuse whose services were well used throughout the week.

In addition to therapeutic sessions, the early Family Camp offered community activities. Because the camp was held during the week of Passover, the entire community prepared and shared in the rituals of the Passover meal. Following the meal, the group attended an "all you can eat sundae festival." A local ice cream shop served the group the world's largest ice cream sundae, prepared on top of a door and carried into the shop by four waiters. Twenty-five years later, Al and Sheila Wild, two veteran campers who attended the early Family Camp, enthusiastically described to us the chaos and mess of eating the sundae as its toppings dripped off the door's sides and onto the floor.

After the first camp, a committee of attendees organized the following year's program, which was again held at Pacific Palisades. While preparing for the second camp, Virginia noticed that many of the original families had registered for a second time. This could provide the opportunity to work with and observe the impact of an intentional community experience on the children, she realized. So, she proposed to the committee that they establish a more formal organization designed to provide mental health practitioners and their families with training as well as develop a community to support families in becoming more fully human. The organizers enthusiastically endorsed this vision and Satir Family Camp (sfc) was born.

Virginia combined aspects of all of her other therapeutic work (including the wilderness camps) into her grandest experiment to date: an intentional community. This vision was the community's entrance into the Definition stage of community development. As the community began, Virginia and the first individuals and families who came to camp defined the premise under which the group continues to work together today: "to become more fully human." Virginia planned the community as a place where people would live and work together in an environment designed to enhance both their emotional and spiritual growth. In all her work, she taught that humans share a life spirit with all other forms of life found on and in the earth. Since 1969, she had been using wilderness camping experiences as a way to enhance that spiritual awareness. She very much wanted to provide a similar experience for members of the sfc.

Nelson's First Day at Camp

After Nelson met Virginia, he and Felix set out to find a place for the family to establish their campsite. It quickly became obvious that people have already claimed many areas. A way up the stream, sheets hung on ropes strung between trees, marking out a large encampment. Felix explained that Virginia and her "inner circle" camped there. Felix suggested that Nelson might want to join another encampment that includes the "young families with little kids." Since the area Felix pointed to is closer to one of the latrines and the showers, it made sense to Phyllis and they set up camp there. Erecting the tent was a challenge. After finally figuring out all the different poles and stakes, Nelson thought he has it done until, in one shuddering moment, the middle pole collapsed and the tent fell into a heap. After a few choice words, Nelson started again with some help from the family setting up near them. Eventually, he stood back to survey his kingdom. He thought, "I sure hope we can keep the damn thing up for seven more days." The significance of this hope was brought home to him as he turned around and saw the last truck chugging back up the mountain.

They spent the rest of the afternoon meeting people and familiarizing themselves with their new environment. Phyllis, ever outgoing, pulled over more and more people for introductions, and Mia was equally successful in making new friends. She enthusiastically introduced her parents to young Adam, who became the family's tour guide. After showing them the key parts of the camp, such as the kitchen and the showers, Adam decided to take Mia to explore the creek. Before they got ten feet away, Phyllis stopped them to insist that Nelson go along. Adam agreed when he realized that Phyllis, like all new moms, would not let Mia go off without an adult.

"Don't worry," Adam told Mia confidentially, "she'll get over it real quick. All moms kind of freak out about us being on our own in the beginning, and then they just realize it's Family Camp and we can take care of ourselves."

As they wandered away from the camp and its ambient noise, the only sound Nelson heard was the splash of water over rock. Suddenly he was struck by a sense of peace he had not felt since he was about Mia's age. He remembered how wonderful it felt to wander unsupervised with his friends, exploring areas he felt no human eye but his had ever seen. Nelson found himself slowing down and letting the kids run off ahead, wanting to give Mia that same sense of freedom.

The Pico Blanco Campsite

As a result of Virginia's connection with a landowner in Big Sur, the camp found Pico Blanco, a setting that proved to have a long and enduring impact on the SFC community. (For views of Pico Blanco, see photos 1–8 in the section before Part Two.)

Pico Blanco is in a remote mountainous area on the coast of northern California. The Big Sur area is generally damp, often immersed in fog, and majestically beautiful in an austere fashion. The section of land used by the camp was at the bottom of a gorge, surrounded by steep hills and redwood trees. The central camping area was a flat area filled with tree stumps and large boulders, with a creek flowing through the middle. Setting up a campsite to meet the basic needs of eighty to a hundred campers for a week required extensive planning and creative jerry-rigging.

The landowners provided much of the camp's logistical support. Trucks transported campers from a central parking area located in a field at the top of Pico Blanco. The camp's limited amenities were also created and maintained by Harry, the camp caretaker and primary fix-it man. A tall, gangly man in his mid-60s when Camp began, Harry was a crusty curmudgeon, according to early campers. It was well known that he considered the whole camp "nuts" but provided many invaluable services nonetheless. He loved to tinker and enjoyed challenges. Maintaining a camp for up to a hundred people in the wilderness of the Big Sur certainly provided just that type of work.

With the assistance of a small group of campers, Harry created a kitchen area for preparing three hot meals a day for the entire camp. Butane gas generators powered the stove and refrigeration unit. Set up against a granite ledge, the area was open air yet could be covered with tarps when it rained. Bob Isles, an early sfc camper, remembered the Pico Blanco kitchen area:

> The appliances were lined up against a steep hillside. It was not straight, but formed something like a French curve. They included four propane refrigerators and freezers at the left end, a series of double sinks with both hot and cold water, at least two commercial propane stoves each with six burners along with a large grill and ovens, then another series of sinks. At the far right end were two one-hundred-gallon propane water heaters, supplying both the kitchen and the showers, which were just beyond them. The showers had three shower heads.
>
> In front of the array of appliances described above was a wooden slatted walkway, about four feet wide. Then separating the appliances from the area where the tables constructed of redwood rounds were, was a large counter, consisting of redwood boards resting on redwood stumps, forming a counter surface. These were used to hold things, to serve food, to serve as cutting boards. At the left end of the counters holes existed into which people inserted Campari umbrellas to protect awaiting food from the sun. They were interrupted in two places by two large double sinks. At the far right end was a bathtub, which served for washing pots and pans, and the occasional infant or toddler. After meals the counter adjacent to the bathtub was set up with tubs to be used for washing personal dishes. This counter was separated from the table area by a walkway that was fairly level, and at the other edge of the walkway was a heavy cable on which our dish bags were hung. The walkway was on one side of the dish bags; the other side dropped down about a foot, marking the area where the sitting area was. The sitting area was perhaps fifteen or twenty feet wide, and edged on the far side by a very large redwood log, one which people would sit. On the far side of this log was the Little Sur River, perhaps twenty feet below the

level of the eating area. The flowing stream provided white noise, which was ubiquitous throughout the camp.

We had inadequate refrigerator space, so produce was spread out on coil bed springs sitting in the edge of the river, keeping it cool. Part of meal preparation was going down to the river to fetch the produce necessary for the meal.

Large redwood stumps originally scattered around the land were moved into the central area near the kitchen. The stumps served as both seats and tables. Each family brought eating utensils and dishes and hung them in bags on cable that surrounded the dining area. The uncovered eating area was chilly, especially in the early morning fog. Nonetheless, this area was the primary gathering and socializing spot at sfc. The cooks knew all the comings and goings and camp gossip because of this location.

The only other amenities provided for campers were showers and latrines. Harry and his crew created the latrines by stringing pipes and hoses into several areas around the camp. The fact that the latrines had five flush toilets located on hillsides, surrounded by sheeting, and open on top just made the whole experience a little more surreal. The communal showers were also open air and, in the spirit of the times, coed.

Tess's Story: Surviving the Latrine

Even with flush toilets and hot and cold showers, Pico Blanco was a primitive area. When the weather changed or illness struck, it was sometimes a very difficult place to be. (See photos 7 and 8 in the section just before Part Two.)

Tess was invited to Satir Family Camp by her friend Alicia. After listening to Alicia's stories about camp every year, Tess finally agreed to attend. Years later, Tess remembered, "I looked forward to camping and having time to spend with Alicia. I really didn't know much about the camp itself, especially where it was located."

The two women drove to the camp together and were greeted enthusiastically upon their arrival in the parking lot. It is clear that Alicia had made many friends over the years and reveled in being among them again. Tess, on the other hand, felt overwhelmed by the size of the group and totally alone among them. More upsetting was her dawning awareness that once she got on the waiting trucks, she would not be able to leave until the following Saturday.

As Tess comprehended that she would be trapped with these people in the wilderness, her tormenting inner voice began to rant: "See, I told you this is a bad idea. It's not just bad, it's stupid. Who do you think you are, coming here and trying to be part of this group? See how much they like Alicia? You think they're going to like you as well? Just wait till they find out what a wimp you are. You're going to be miserable. Just look at the gear other people brought. You don't have the right stuff. You're probably going to freeze, and your tent will collapse, and no one will care one bit."

While talking to Tess, Alicia was getting her gear ready. Tess could hear Alicia speaking but was so panicked that she did not comprehend the words. Just as Tess got up the nerve to tell Alicia that she just could not go, a voice cried out, "Okay, Satir Family Campers, the truck is ready. Let's load up and get going."

Alicia picked up her gear and cheerfully motioned for Tess to follow. As awful as Tess felt about going to camp, she felt even worse about stopping Alicia from going. Trapped in this conflict, she let herself be swept onto the truck with about ten laughing people. Worried about being sick on the ride down the mountain, she sat on the end and clung to the rail, hoping maybe she would just fall off and end the whole dilemma.

But she did not, and by the end of the ride was overtaken by the beauty and majesty of Pico Blanco. Once she accepted that there would be no escape, she submitted to the energy of her fellow passengers. When the truck stopped at the main camping area, Tess had begun to convince herself it would not be so bad. The beauty of the place pleased her, and her love of the outdoors and camping provided some balance to her fear and panic about dealing with such a large number of new people. As Alicia's friend, Tess obtained immediate acceptance, and as long as Alicia was with her, she could relax.

That state quickly dissipated on her tour of the "facilities." Although the latrines are flush toilets, Tess found something bizarre about sitting on a flush toilet in an area open to the elements, even if she was surrounded by plastic sheeting. It got worse when Tess realized that the showers are coed. As always, Alicia came to her rescue on the second day, when they showered together and she showed Tess the privacy sign, which alerted others to Tess's desire to shower alone. Tess again relaxed. By the end of her second day, although not happy, she felt she could endure.

Tess found the therapy sessions (what sfc calls "work sessions") fascinating. She envied the courage of people who chose to address their issues in front of the group. By observing others work, she learned a great deal about Virginia Satir's methods and about her own issues. She became particularly aware of how "The Inner Critic" had been affecting her life.

Informal times around camp are much more challenging, however. Tess had the most difficulty when Alicia was not around to serve as a buffer. Without her best friend, she sat alone and tried to look as if she were content with the solitude. Several times when campers joined her, she became tongue-tied by her lack of confidence. She participated in the introductory part of the social discourse, responding to questions such as: "Where are you from?", "How did you hear about camp?", "How long have you known Alicia?" When it came to questions such as "How do you like camp?" or "What did you think of the session?", however, Tess found it difficult to articulate her thoughts and ideas. She had a lot to say, but most of her responses stayed bottled inside. When these awkward conversations ended and the person left, Tess's Inner Critic weighed in: "Well, you made a great impression. What a stupid remark you made. That person must think you are a total idiot. Did you see how quickly she left to talk to someone else? No wonder no one ever wants to sit with you. The only reason they put up with you is 'cause you're Alicia's friend. Who do you think you are to come here and pretend like you are some capable therapist? You are just the same worthless little girl who will never grow up."

Following these interactions, Tess often rushed away to the comfort of her tent. When she again retreated to her tent on the third day, she realized she did not feel well. Assuming the feeling was just part of her panic, she willed away the upset in her stomach. By evening, however, she could no longer ignore her discomfort. Tess had contracted a flu bug, complete with vomiting and diarrhea, that was passing through the whole camp. Alicia came to console Tess the next day, assuring her that most people were up and about after 24 hours. By that time, Tess was spending all her energy trying to get to and from the latrine. She and Alicia had the misfortune of camping in an area where the closest latrine was directly up a hill.

"After what felt like the fiftieth time I crawled up that hill, I lay there knowing I was never going to get home. I just knew I would die right there on that hill, trying to get to a damn latrine in the middle of nowhere."

Instead of dying, Tess reached the latrine and returned to her tent. By the end of the second day, she began to feel better. That night, tired and weak, she once again joined the communal activities to get some food. Because camp ran only one more day, Tess did little more than go to meals and sleep. When the trucks arrived to return the campers to the parking lot, she wearily packed up and was one of the first to climb on for the trip out. Talking about that experience years later, Tess remembered:

> As I rode up out of the canyon I felt like I was leaving the darkness and entering the light. When I got into my car, I burst into tears. I was so glad to be free of that place. I knew that I could never return. I felt like it was a miracle that I had survived and I found no redeeming value in the suffering that I had experienced. Right then and there, I promised that I would never allow myself to suffer like that again.

For most others who attended SFC at Pico Blanco, the primitive nature of the area was a large part of the attraction. Campsites were left to the ingenuity of each family. Virginia had the largest encampment, affectionately known as the "The Pleasure Palace." Although most of the camping areas were on the hillsides, campers usually found some spot of level ground on which to pitch their tents. Tents and sometimes encampments of several tents were scattered along the stream's banks. Parallel to the stream was a rutted dirt path that served as the camp road, running from the central kitchen area at one end to the amphitheater at the other. Created in a grove of redwood trees, the amphitheater consisted of a small plot of flat ground where Virginia demonstrated her theories by working with individuals and families. Members of the camp sat and observed the work on chairs spread around the clearing or perched precariously on the hillside.

Pico Blanco Campers

Most of the early SFC campers came from California although some participants attended from other states and other countries. Participants included families in the broadest sense of the word and divided loosely into two groups. At the early camps, when Virginia was the leader, one group was composed of professional therapists who had personal or professional ties to Virginia. Most of these campers came because of their connection with her. Some of these members did not have children and attended either as single individuals or with partners. During the Virginia years, this group became known as the "Inner Circle." Membership in this group occurred in different ways at camp. Some members were family therapists who worked with Virginia during the year. Others were Virginia's clients or personal friends. Some campers joined the Inner Circle by being invited to camp near Virginia or to sit with her at meals or during free time.

The owners of the Pico Blanco land also attended and had special privileges. During camp, Virginia and the owners sometimes took a break from camp living and went up to the top of the mountain to spend time with Harry and his wife, Marta, who camped in a house trailer that had all the amenities of daily life. Select campers were also invited to visit and partake of Marta's famous pies. Campers who received such invitations were also seen as part of the Inner Circle, at least for that year. As one female camper related:

> It was interesting that almost all of Virginia's "favorites" at camp were men. She would spend time with the men and just ignore their wives or partners. I don't know of any woman from our group who got invited to have Marta's pies. Even though my husband was one of Virginia's favorites, he began to avoid her because he resented the way she always acted like I wasn't even present when she spent time with us.

In general, the second group comprised parents with young children who learned about camp by having either attended one of Virginia's trainings during the year or through other contact with Virginia's work (such as academic study). Although one person in the couple generally had a connection with the mental health profession, they both were usually not known to Virginia either professionally or personally. In contrast to the Inner Circle, these families chose to return camp each year because of the connections they developed with other young families. The "young families" group found the experience of wilderness camping freeing for themselves and their children. They developed strong bonds and connections with each other through the therapeutic work they shared. It is people in this second group who, more than twenty-five years later, are now SFC's senior members. Their children will be the parents of the next generation of young families.

Carl and Sherry

Carl, Sherry, and their two children, Julia and Joey, came to SFC the same year as Nelson and Phyllis. At the hospital where Carl was completing his psychiatric residency, his colleague Sean had told him about the camp. The idea of learning family therapy from Virginia while having a week's vacation with his family intrigued him. With written directions and very little information about what to expect, Carl and Sherry packed the two kids and all their gear into their 1979 Kharmann Ghia and made the long drive to Big Sur, California. Sherry had rueful memories of that first year:

> When I look back now, I realize we did not have a clue what we were getting into. I thought we were going camping with other families. I was just glad to have a whole week where Carl would not be studying or going to the hospital.

Carl remembered the first challenge was to find the place. Their orientation letter made it clear that campers needed to arrive on time or they would miss the truck. Otherwise, their camping trip would end before it even started. Thinking they had plenty of time, the family meandered along, making the many stops required when traveling with young children. To their chagrin, they arrived in Big Sur and the general location of where they thought they would find the camp with little time to spare. Looking at the map, they circled around the land and finally came upon a road with a sign: "Welcome to Satir Family Camp."

Driving into the parking lot, they got an enthusiastic greeting from the Welcoming Committee and received their Satir Family Camp tee shirts. They had arrived about fifteen minutes after the scheduled departure time and soon learned that timeliness was not going to be a big issue at camp.

As they unloaded their gear and milled around meeting other campers, Carl and Sherry noticed a family near them struggling to organize what looked their entire collection of household belongings. "Well," thought Carl, "I sure am glad I convinced Sherry to leave those other suitcases at home. And they only have one kid with them! That poor guy."

Shortly after, Sherry brought Nelson and Phyllis over to introduce Carl. Nelson's self-deprecating humor charmed Carl. Phyllis and Sherry sorted the vast belongings into a manageable pile while Carl helped Nelson repack the non-essentials back into Nelson's car. Finally, the truck they were all awaiting drove up from behind the parking lot. Carl, Sherry, and the two children piled onto the truck's benches. "Hang on tight," yelled Harry, their driver, and off they went on the infamous ride down Pico Blanco and into the gully. All around them, people laughed and called out greetings. After some initial anxiety—heightened by low-hanging tree limbs, the speed of the ride, and several hairpin curves—Carl and Sherry got into the swing of things.

Although struck by the majesty of their surroundings, both Carl and Sherry were slightly overwhelmed by the realities of camping with very young children in such a primitive place. Unbeknownst to them, Joey was the youngest child in the group. As they unloaded their belongings, they watched the many adults and older children clambering about. Sherry looked with anxiety at the flowing stream and wondered how on earth she would keep Joey safe, never mind clean and dry, for a week. Carl also began to wonder if they had made a mistake in coming.

His colleague Sean called from across the stream, "Welcome you two, come and meet some of the campers!" Once Carl and Sherry found a place to cross the stream, Sean introduced them to Felix, who responded to Carl's handshake with a masculine embrace. Felix laughed and said, "Don't worry, you'll get use to it. Virginia finally convinced me that hugs really are the best way to say hello. You know, hugs are necessary for survival and growth."

Carl shared a skeptical glance with Nelson but allowed himself to get caught up in the warmth and caring expressed by the many new people they were meeting. Several older children came up and offered to show Julia around. Another asked if she could play with Joey while Carl and Sherry set up camp. After a slight hesitancy, Sherry let them both go and turned with Carl to follow Sean and his wife Wanda who volunteered to help them find a good place to set up camp. Wanda suggested they might want to be near the "facilities" while casually pointing out to a sheeted area they were passing.

"There's the shower. We're pretty casual around here. Most people shower with whomever arrives at the same time. If that's a problem, just put out the privacy sign and you can shower alone. I started out that way, but after a while it just seemed natural to shower whenever and with whomever. You may feel differently, with the kids and all. You just decide what is best for you."

"Okay," thought Sherry. "I can just see me and the kids and all these people in the shower together. I wonder if we can change our minds and go home." Carl looked at her, gave her a wink and a smile, and they kept on walking.

"Over here," suggested Sean, pointing up the hillside to where a relatively flat area spread among several trees.

"It's pretty flat, and you can run a rope between the trees for a clothesline. Not that stuff dries real well around here, but you can try.

"Now, the latrines are over there." He pointed in a direction of the clump of trees that Wanda had already showed them. "I know it looks primitive," he said consolingly, "but they are honest-to-god flush toilets in there."

Sherry thought, "This will really set back Joey's potty training. Thank goodness, I brought his potty chair. In fact, maybe I'll just use it myself now and then, especially if it rains, which it sure feels like right now." Turning to Wanda, she inquired casually, "What do you do if it rains?"

"Oh, don't even think about rain," Wanda responded in mock horror. "We just do a lot of sun dances, and if it happens, we usually survive." With that, Wanda said her good-byes so that she could go and greet new arrivals.

Carl saw that Nelson and Phyllis had selected a site next to them. Sean, Nelson, and Carl set up Carl's tent while Phyllis and Sherry shared information about kids and how they got connected to Family Camp. Finally, Sean instructed Carl and Sherry on where to put their dishes before setting off with a cheerful wave and departing comment: "Take your time getting set up. You'll hear a bell about 6:30, and that means dinner is ready. Let's sit together tonight. If you brought beer, by the way, just stick it in the creek and it will stay pretty cold." He pointed to an area where several six-packs were floating. "Natural refrigeration, isn't it great?"

Pico Blanco Programs

The early SFC was organized by a loose group of participants who became known as "the Committee." The Committee took over the tasks originally performed by Jackie Schwartz. Prior to each annual camp, they met quarterly to plan the program, handle organizational issues, and review new camper applications. They also coordinated logistics, down to the minute details of who brought which kitchen utensil. They held their final meeting before camp at Pico Blanco so the Committee could help prepare the site.

SFC's organizational structure grew slowly. The Committee collected camper fees, paid Virginia for her services, and paid the owners for use of their land. The self-selected camp registrar and secretary kept the camp minutes. During this period, agreements and understandings were written down, but in general the camp thrived on its informality and commitment to process versus outcome.

The Committee was responsible for planning the family events for each annual camp. In addition to daily Temperature Readings (described fully in Chapter 8) and work sessions with Virginia, the entire camp could join in special events, such as climbing to the top of the mountain, fishing, and hiking to the swimming hole or to the ocean. Over the years, other activities included a party known as White Night, where campers dressed in white for a formal party in the wilderness; Skit Night, where local talent performed for the entire camp; and a "crazy tee shirt lunch" (Wagner, 1987, p. 10).

The Children at Pico Blanco

Virginia viewed children as equal participants in the community and insisted on including them in all the activities. Sherry learned about this philosophy when she raised her worries about Joey at her first Temperature Reading.

Virginia: Sherry, you have a bug?

Sherry: Well, it's more like a concern.

Virginia: Okay, what can we help you with?

Sherry: Well, I can't figure out how I'm going to come to sessions.

Virginia [*looking puzzled*]: Because . . . ?

Sherry: It's Joey. See, I know Julia will be okay, because she is playing with other kids and can come find me if she needs anything; but Joey just turned three, and ———

Virginia [*interrupting with a confident air*]: Well, Sherry, you just need to trust that Joey will take care of himself. Now, you want to be sure that he knows where you are and show him how to get to the amphitheater when you are there. But, I assure you, Joey will take care of himself.

Many years later when Sherry shared this story, she laughed while reporting:

> And you know what, that's just what I did. I took Joey to the sessions and for a while, he would sit with me. Then he would wander off, and I just trusted that he would take care of himself. When I think about it now, I'm amazed I did that. I mean, there was a creek of running water down the middle of the campsite, and he had just turned three!

But when Virginia said it, it just made sense, and I was able to let go. I know a lot of the older girls played with him, but there was no one actually responsible for watching him. I don't think I could do that today. Eventually, the camp did develop a program for the little children; but that first year, Joey was part of camp like all the big kids, and he really did take care of himself, just like Virginia said he would!

As more families with young children joined camp, as mentioned, pressure arose to organize activities for the younger children. The Children's Program was thus initiated. At least one adult, assisted by the older children, organized and offered activities for young children while their parents were in work sessions.

Attending Satir Family Camp was an intense experience, so Virginia and the Committee continued to schedule a free day on Wednesdays. In addition to giving campers a break from the camp's therapeutic aspects, she added the concept of a Free University day. Each Wednesday, people could share their interests, knowledge, and expertise with other campers. Both the Children's Program and the Free University day continue as parts of annual sfc activities.

Therapeutic Programs

During the years that Virginia was at camp, the therapeutic program consisted of daily Temperature Readings, which involved the entire community; didactic trainings, often given as meditations at the Temperature Readings; and work sessions. Virginia was in complete charge of the program. She facilitated each Temperature Reading, and she decided what topics to present at the trainings, what issues to address, and who would do work in the formal therapy sessions.

Virginia's simplest yet most powerful technique was her use of self. Campers who worked with Virginia describe her personality as "larger than life." Others speak of her "magic," her gift for saying the right thing at just the right moment. Campers describe her eyes as "the blue headlights" and speak of feeling almost frozen in place when she looked at them. Those who knew her also speak of how, when she was working with them or addressing them as an individual, she made them each feel like the only person in her universe.

Her physical presence was imposing. She was a tall, large-boned woman who easily dominated a group simply by being present. She also used touch to connect with others, often holding hands or putting an arm around the person with whom she was working. She

encouraged physical contact with others and believed that "all people need a daily minimum of four hugs for physical survival, eight
hugs for maintenance, and twelve hugs for growth" (Bonar, 2004).

In addition, Virginia had great verbal skills. She told stories and
utilized creative metaphors and gentle humor to illustrate her work as
well as to soothe tension or emotions that arose during the work. Her
meditations were full of descriptions used to bring groups together. She
also used body awareness to help people concentrate and incorporate
the knowledge she had to share. Virginia continually stressed the connections between people in families as well as in communities. She
often used ropes to help people visualize these connections. When
talking about Virginia, campers universally mention the omnipresent
rope that Virginia kept around her waist so that whenever a situation
arose, she could demonstrate how people are connected.

She also believed in the connection between people and the
earth. She continually turned to the camp's natural setting to help
members connect with themselves and with each other. Virginia's
spirituality is particularly evident in her meditations, as shown in her
meditation at a workshop in 1983 (Satir & Banmen, 1984, pp. 1–2):

> . . . And let yourself further become aware that your feet, resting
> on the floor, are not only supported by the floor, but by the energy that
> comes from the center of the universe, coming up through your feet
> and legs and into your body, giving you your source of groundedness. . . .
> This energy is forever available for people through the day, all day
> long, all of the time that you live and breathe on this planet. . . .
> [You need only] your awareness to be in touch, and . . . take
> advantage of that energy. Energy of groundedness that comes
> from the center of the earth.
>
> Let yourself become aware of the energy from the heavens, as it
> moves down through the top of your head into your face and neck,
> arms and chest, meeting the energy of groundedness. . . . That energy
> from the heavens, the energy of inspiration, of sensing, of
> imagination, the place where all the real imaging is grounded. And as
> the energy of intuition, inspiration, of sensing meets the energy of
> groundedness, it forms still a third energy. And the energy of
> intuition, imagination, and sensing is also forever there. It waits only
> for you to acknowledge access to it.
>
> And as these two energies mingle together, the third energy they
> create is the energy of connectedness with another human being, the
> energy that flows out through your arms and skin and eyes, facial
> expression, to other persons, creating the bonding, the joy, the
> possibilities of building with other people. . . .

During the years that Virginia led camp, the psychological work often "bubbled up" out of daily events. When individuals expressed concerns about an issue in camp, Virginia looked for the deeper issue expressed within that concern, believing that all strong reactions or concerns stem from family-of-origin issues. When someone reacted with intensity, was unable to hear different points of view, or hung onto his or her point of view almost without reason, Virginia stopped the discussion, called the person to the front of the group, and began a work session. Her abilities to read a person's readiness to work seemed almost magical, but her formative years had taught her to pay close attention to the nonverbal cues of those on whom she depended for her survival needs.

Who Gets to Work

Virginia also knew when people were not ready to work, as illustrated in the following story by Meredith.

> At age 35, Fred had already moved through four different careers. Time after time, he took a job only to decide within a few months that "it doesn't offer enough stimulation" or "there is no one at my level for me to grow with." At camp, he was always seeking out Virginia's attention. From the day he arrived, he continually asked if he could work on "finding his niche." Virginia's quiet but firm response was, "You aren't ready yet. You need to yeast and find out what it is you really want to work on."

Arriving for his third camp with his wife, Meredith, and their two daughters, Fred described to anyone who would listen his job woes. He repeatedly expressed his desire to work on how to find the right place for his skills and interests. Meredith came to camp with feelings of quiet desperation. Fred had just left yet another secure job with a decent if modest paycheck and benefits for the whole family. She was once again the family's sole source of financial support. Fred's decision left her trapped in a secretarial job at a time when she had hoped to return to school to develop her own professional interests. She fervently wished that Virginia would allow Fred to work, hoping that the work might help him actually find a job and keep it.

Over their time at camp, Meredith had quietly watched as Virginia selected people to work. She gradually recognized that Virginia almost never chose people who came to camp "wanting to work." Meredith suspected that Virginia understood that these people were not wanting to do work; rather, they were looking for some magic to solve their problems. "That is exactly what Fred does," Meredith mused. "He is always looking for some magic that will help him avoid doing the hard work."

Camp for Meredith and Fred went as usual that year. At every Temperature Reading, Fred sat in the front row, avidly trying to catch Virginia's eye. He talked constantly to anyone who would listen, which eventually caused people to avoid his company.

Meredith, on the other hand, spent more and more time with her group of women friends. She attended work sessions when she could but spent most of her time with the kids so that Fred could attend every session. It was therefore a total surprise when, at the end of Temperature Reading on Thursday, Virginia asked Meredith to come up to the front. With great trepidation, she went forward and stood next to Virginia.

> I remember feeling this great tall warmth standing beside me. When Virginia took my hands in hers and turned me to look in her eyes, I felt like all this weight came off me and the tears just began to slide down my face. Then I heard Virginia say; "I think it is time for you to find out what is behind all those tears. Will you be willing to work with me this afternoon?"

This story is just one example of Virginia's great skill at identifying when a person was ready or not ready to do work. Using this skill, Virginia made sure that people who worked at camp were prepared to use the work for their personal growth and that the work would benefit the community as well as the individual.

Campers' Views of SFC During the Pico Blanco Years

During SFC's tenth year and two years following Virginia's departure, Judith Wagner conducted research and published the results in her thesis, *"The Effects of Satir Family Camp on Individuals and Their Families: A Qualitative Study"* (1987). A camper during the Pico Blanco years, she recorded interviews with five families (nine adults and their eight children, ages 8–13) who at that time had attended SFC from four to six years. Wagner asked the adults and children about Virginia and the therapeutic work done at camp. The following quotes are from their responses (Wagner, 1987, pp. 26–28).

> The primary contribution of Virginia is what she has taught us about communication and being in the present and expressing ourselves and her Family Reconstruction. [—A father]

Virginia's contributions were substantial. Personally, I learned so much every time she did a piece of work that it was virtually unthinkable not to be there. . . . Virginia touched peoples' hearts and souls very quickly. . . . I felt people became too reliant on wanting to go to this one person [Virginia] and have her transform everything like the magician waving her wand . . . forgetting that the power to be transformed rests within each of us. That's what Virginia has been trying to teach them, camp after camp after camp. [—A father]

. . . I thought of her as a gifted violinist, she was an artist. I was amazed at her ability to listen. . . . Virginia set up a structure; she built a space where it could happen. She gave us a vision so that we knew it was important for it to happen. [—A mother]

Virginia had a vision. Her principle and boldness to even try family therapy [in a camp setting] . . . including all the different types of non-conventional families . . . a woman before her time. . . . her love and concern are quite evident and for me, her power and intelligence—she's human, don't get me wrong, she does have her human frailties like anybody else, but her love and caring just exude from her. I like her style. She is a Grand Dame. [—A mother]

She set the tone of it being a safe place and having good vibes. People were there not to hurt but help each other. There was something real that went on there that didn't occur outside. She was the one who called the shots. They were her rules. I remember most not only her sense of humor, but also her meditations. I remember the last one she did very well—what a gift that was. . . .[—A mother]

The following quotes from Wagner's interviews describe how the children viewed their experiences with Virginia.

I think Virginia did a lot. She helped with therapy and helped other people with their problems. She tried many ways to work their problems out. When she's there, I try to talk to her. [—Male, age 11]

She was always trying to work out problems that people had. . . some people would be fighting and having grudges. [—Female, age 9]

Yeah, I remember her but I didn't see her work a lot. She was really an interesting person. I could never quite figure her out. There were a lot of levels of her. . . I like her a lot. She was neat, very smart. I saw her different from the other adults there. [—Female, age 13]

I remember Virginia real well. I remember that she liked most everybody. She always had a smiling face. . . . Not very many big speeches since Virginia left. [—Male, age 11]

Wagner also asked the children to describe their experiences with children and families at camp.

. . . I think people who go to camp are more aware of certain things like feelings. . . . It's weird that I've only known some of them for only four weeks out of my life and I probably know them better than just about everybody else that I've gone to school with my entire life. [—Female, age 11]

When asked if they saw more or less of their family at camp, various children responded:

No, I don't think so because we're all living in the same house at home and at camp we all have our own tents and different things and activities to do. . . . I feel close [to my family]. . . . Some of the time I talk to my brother. At home we talk a lot, but some of it's fighting and that's not good. We hardly ever do any fighting at camp. . . . I think it's that we have a lot more things to do at camp. When my brother doesn't have anything to do, he picks on me at home. So I like camp. . . . I think my parents are happy at camp because they have a lot of friends to talk to. They can go to therapy and meetings and they can do a lot of things without worrying about me and my brother. [—Female, age 9]

All our other vacations we are with them [our parents] all the time, while at camp it's more realistic. . . . My brother is with his friends and I'm with my friends which makes it more fulfilling to be together, going to the meetings together. You can experience what you want, you don't have to do what your parents want you to do, which is really good. . . . Part of the family is letting you be who your are . . . [Our parents are] more happy. They're more willing to let me have fun my way. [—Female, age 13]

Sometimes [I see them] less because I like doing new things there like hiking and being free. You sign up for kitchen duty and I like the cooking part. . . . I see my sister and my parents a little bit, but we pretty much stay with our own friends. . . . My parents are happy unless something big happens that's a big mistake. I think they're happy there most of the time. . . . It's fun [to have your own tent] because your mom can tuck you in, but then you're on your own. One time I thought my tent was slipping down [the hill] but it was fine. [—Male, age 11]

When asked whether they would encourage their future families to attend sfc when they are grown, all but one of the children said yes. The one child who did not envision attending as an adult predicted, "It wouldn't be around" (Wagner, 1987, p. 34).

Other children discussed what they would tell their families about attending camp:

> I'd tell [my future husband] it was great, the food was wonderful because by then I'd probably like lasagna and all those vegetables. If he likes skits, I'd tell him that there's lots of neat skits at the end. . . . I'd tell my kids that there's lots of kids there they can play with and have fun with, and I went there since I was three. [—Female, age 9]
>
> I would say that it's fun and you get to meet new people. People cook for you and you don't have to cook. You can relax the whole time. [—Male, age 11]
>
> I'd tell [my future wife] there will be lots of fun things. There'd be showers, bathrooms and baths. There's lots of people to talk to. She'd probably like to take the experience. [—Male, age 8]

Several of these children continue to attend camp and were interviewed again for this book, along with other young adults who have attended camp throughout their childhood. Their memories of being young children at camp continue to be positive. The young woman who was first interviewed at age 9 talked to the author about how different her experience had been from that of the boys.

> I remember [the boys] just hung out in this fort they created on the hillside. They would go up there and paint themselves and carry sticks and stuff. It was kind of a scene out of *Lord of the Flies*. Finally it got out of control and had to be shut down. Boy, did that take a lot of time to process.

When asked what she was doing while the boys were playing in the fort, she responded:

> Oh, the girls were a lot tamer. I remember I used to get my face painted and we just kind of played with each other . . . little girl stuff. We weren't allowed in the fort, which made me mad.

Another of the children interviewed by Wagner now brings his family to camp. He told us of his experience growing up at SFC.

> I started to go to camp when I was two, so I really don't have any memories of *not* being at camp. I guess I'm unique 'cause I've gone from being a child to a teen to a young adult, and this year I'm here as a parent. My first real memories of camp are at Pico Blanco. We used to jump on these mattresses in the back of the amphitheater. That is

my whole sense of being a kid at camp . . . being able to do things you could never do at home. I mean, we would spend hours jumping on those mattresses 'cause who could jump on the beds at home? We just tore those suckers apart! There was so much freedom at Pico Blanco. We could go off in the woods or play in the creek. And it just seemed there were never adults around, just us kids.

I wasn't too much involved in the therapy stuff as a kid. I *hated* Temperature Reading. It was so boring listening to grownups talk all the time. But at least we had trees to climb and then they put the mattresses in the back and we had something to do. I did like the Appreciations part. I always counted up how many appreciations I got. It was like a goal to get the highest number of any kid. I think I did that till I was about 12. And it wasn't just a game. Getting "warm fuzzies" [the affectionate term used at camp for appreciative statements] meant a lot when I was little.

The best part for me as a kid, though, was the fort we built on the hill at Pico Blanco. Each kid . . . well, boys, actually 'cause no girls were allowed, except to visit, maybe. Anyway, each kid built his own section. I was pretty little, so mine wasn't much. But Kevin, he must have been about 12, he had a part we called "Kevin's Castle."

We had lots of branches and rocks. We were always looking for stuff to put in our fort. Each year, we added more and more. That was the first thing you did when you got to camp. You rushed up the hill to check out the fort and see what was left from last year.

Then one year, we kind of got carried away. It really was kind of *Lord of the Flies* at that point. We started to have this system where we piled up rocks like we were going to war. Now, this was on a hillside, so all these rocks were piled up and just held back by sticks. Then one day somebody pulled out the sticks and the rocks just poured down the hill. It was really scary, and some of the little kids actually got hurt by the rocks. And then the fort became a really big deal. Man, the adults talked for hours about what happened, what we were doing, and all that stuff. Kind of took the fun out of the fort after that, 'cause the grownups were always checking us out.

The fort experience was not the only event that created stress and long process sessions during the years at Pico Blanco. As described earlier, adults sometimes became very concerned and often unhappy during the camp experience. One of these events, mentioned by almost everyone who camped during the Pico Blanco years, is the "the snake incident." The following story recounts that event, although the dialogue and names of campers are fictional.

The Snake Incident

On Wednesday of the Year of the Snake Incident, a large group of campers, including a number of children, went on a hike to the top of Pico Blanco. As usual, Harry led the hike. Just as they reached the summit, Harry called out, "Watch the kids!"

Phyllis grabbed Joey's hand and looked around for Mia. With relief, she saw Nelson waving at her and realized that he was surrounded by Mia, Julia, and Adam. Sherry came up behind Phyllis and asked, "What is Harry doing?"

"No idea," replied Phyllis, "but I figure if Harry says, 'Grab the kids,' we'd better beware."

Sure enough, just as everyone gathered, a huge bang resounded. All the kids ran toward the sound. The adults were close on their heels. Phyllis and Sherry found Harry in the middle of the group, holding a gun in one hand and a huge snake in the other. When the parents got over their initial shock, Phyllis asked Harry: "Did you really have to shoot it?"

In an irritated tone, Harry replied, "Of course. Did you want it to bite Mia? It's a rattler, and they do bite, you know."

At that point, Nelson moved in behind Phyllis and put his hand on her shoulder. Phyllis wasn't sure if he wanted her to be quiet or to stand up to Harry, but she goes ahead, knowing she is taking a risk. She tells Harry, "To be honest, I'm more worried about a loaded gun around Mia than a snake."

Several other parents then joined the conversation. Fred, the most dominant voice, said, "Oh, let's not have a big discussion, okay? It's done and over with. Harry already put his gun away, so let's just finish the hike."

With that, the group turned away from Phyllis and continued hiking to the mountaintop.

Years later, campers shared different perspectives about the Snake Incident and about what caused the upheaval at camp. Jerry, the cook, remembers the event as an educational opportunity for the children. During the evening, the snake's skin was displayed for all to see. Several of the campers that year were biologists and provided an impromptu lesson on rattlesnakes. Jerry prepared snake meat for anyone willing to try a new epicurean delight. He described the event: "As far as I was concerned, it was a good night after a tense day. Yeah, Harry went a little overboard shooting the damned thing. I would have just hit it with a stick."

Fred described the ensuing concern as typical of how things happened at Family Camp. "All of a sudden, everyone had an opinion about what should have been done. Some people felt the snake should have been left alone. Others were glad we got rid of it. People just went on and on about the rights of all living creatures. The whole thing was *not* worth the discussion it took at camp."

Everyone who remembered the event agreed that it was a big issue for camp and could have caused major fissures among campers were it not for Virginia's skill in working with the community. For her, this event, like everything else that happened at camp, became a point of learning and growth for the community. She was aware that people were upset by the event. As people talked among themselves, the discomfort increased. There was also an undercurrent of dismay about how Harry reacted.

It became clear the community was beginning to divide between those who felt it was appropriate to kill the snake and those who felt the snake deserved to be treated as an equal on the land. As a member of the Committee said, "The Snake Incident just underscored to most of us that camp was only here because the owners chose to let us be here and if we disagreed with them we risked being thrown off the land."

A good part of the camp supported Harry's right to decide what needed to happen on the property and felt the snake supporters were carrying "the back-to-nature stuff" to an extreme. By Thursday morning, the drama created by the Snake Incident was consuming camp. People began to gather at tables, and the tension increased as several discussions erupted into heated arguments. When someone announced it was time for Temperature Reading, the community gathered together slowly to process the event under Virginia's calm leadership.

Campers recall that Temperature Reading as being an endless and sometimes pointless discussion about nature and snakes and who has the right to decide what lives and dies. Interestingly, most people remember only discussing different views regarding the snake. When asked about the gun and its use around the children, the majority of campers who were interviewed agreed that some campers felt concerned but emphasized that no one disagreed openly with actions of Harry or the landlord.

The Snake Incident is just one of many episodes in which the community may have processed a presenting issue without addressing underlying concerns. This pattern contributed to the camp's ongoing denial of inappropriate behavior by a few adult campers. For many years, this behavior remained hidden and unmentioned. It took Virginia's leaving sfc and the camp's relocating from private land before the community addressed these unspoken concerns.

Another example of unaddressed issues at the early sfc is the dichotomy between the Inner Circle or privileged few and the other campers. Although rules and expectations were not always overt, the expectation from Virginia and the group collective was to go along with Virginia's unwritten rules of privilege. In the camp's later years, the formerly unspoken dissatisfaction with some members of the privileged group and their behavior around camp became expressed. The community addressed this in a variety of ways, such as adopting more structure and rules, confronting issues directly or ignoring them, and creating duties and roles. Choosing among these depended on many aspects of camp structure, such as its location, Virginia's presence, and the formal systems of authority and rules of the world outside of camp.

A dichotomy existed within Virginia's role in the early camp's governance. Much of her theory and philosophy rests on her belief in the intrinsic value of every individual based on their value as a being rather than on their status. When she discussed this belief, she often spoke out against organizations that based value on a person's place within the hierarchy. Yet the early camp governance had a strict hierarchy, with Virginia at the top, followed by her Inner Circle. Although the Committee also existed, Virginia ran Family Camp. Her decisions were final and not open to discussion or interpretation. As one Committee member said:

> I guess Virginia was kind of a tyrant, but she was a benevolent tyrant and gave us so much that it was just easier to go along with her. To be honest, there weren't that many things we disagreed with Virginia about. She was such an extraordinary leader that it wasn't hard to give up our autonomy for her wisdom.

Relinquishing alternatives extended farther. Other Committee members said:

> Virginia always let us know that it was her way or not at all. The few times someone disagreed with her, she was clear that she just would not come back if we did not do what she wanted. That kind of operated for the owners of the land at Pico Blanco, too. They also made it clear that if we didn't go along with their decisions, than we

would have to leave the land. After a couple of those discussions, people just stopped expressing any disagreement.

Virginia ran the show, and we all knew it. We also knew that we were camping on private land and that the owners had the final say because Virginia always backed them when they made decisions about the camp and the property. We didn't all like it. Right at the beginning, I even proposed to some friends that we have camp somewhere else so we would be less vulnerable to the owners, but we knew we would never find a place as wonderful as Pico Blanco, so we just adjusted.

Community Implications

The early years at Pico Blanco are ripe with free-flowing form and a general lack of boundaries. The camp's wilderness setting also forced the community to begin its development in a very primitive state. This clearly was Virginia's design, at least in some part. She seemed to want to experiment with the idea and ideal of what a community might amount to over time after developing in an isolated location with few formal boundaries. The connection to the earth, as evidenced in many of her meditations, as well as the desire to locate the camp in a beautiful yet primitive setting appear to be part of a grand design to help people focus on what is important by literally leaving behind the trappings of everyday life. In fact, Pico Blanco served this purpose so well that when the camp was finally forced to relocate in later years, the effect was significant.

sfc's need to focus on basic survival in the wilderness complicated its development as a community. The wilderness environment forced campers to work together and contribute to both the survival and growth of the whole community. During the stages of Definition and Establishment, the community was successful as long as no significant challenges arose to its common goal and its ability to foster coexistence among campers. When a significant challenge arose, such as a foreign viewpoint or a crisis, leaders emerged to direct the group in different directions to alleviate the stress or threat to the common purpose. In the early years, sfc developed in spurts, reacting to different stressors and threats to the prevailing status quo.

It is interesting to consider how events described in this chapter shaped the evolution of sfc. Consistent with the Definition stage, a few influential leaders made most of the decisions. Virginia and a few close allies established the camp's premise, rules, and operations. Campers deferred to the leaders, who presented ideas and had the resources to implement them. Roles of leader and follower were set, and the rules—informal and often unspoken—allowed the community to operate.

In the Establishment stage, the community had to focus first on creating a safe physical environment. After that, enough security prevailed among the campers and within the leadership that the community's energy moved to maintain the status quo as defined by self-selected camp leaders.

During the period of Status Quo, challenges arose regarding the privileged positions held by some campers and the duality of the landlord–camper role. These and other such issues challenged the community and created some of its greatest growth. The Snake Incident is an early example of how a foreign element created new energy in the community. In reaction to the foreign element, the snake, campers began to challenge the status quo of decisions made by a privileged few. Out of this event and the community processing that followed, a new energy emerged and pushed the community toward the stage of Rebellion.

The way that children were supervised during the early years at Pico Blanco is another example of how a new energy, chaos, led to a new stage of community development. The boundaries around child care were loose and open to interpretation during that time. Clearly, Virginia believed that children could be left to their own designs to take what they needed from the camp experience. She encouraged parents to pursue their own agendas and allow their children to grow unencumbered in this setting. This seemed to work fine for a while, but the lack of restrictions and supervision eventually yielded consequences. The boys' stockpiling of rocks as weapons and subsequent injury to some children revealed the energy of chaos that was operating among the children.

The community responded by immediately imposing structure on the children's experience. The boys' actions and subsequent chaotic energy upset the balance of the status quo, which held that the children could manage their freedom at Pico Blanco. The reality of the chaos that can develop when children have no structure also nudged the camp forward.

These two examples illustrate how the early camp usually developed: in reaction to a crisis arising from a lack of boundaries within the community. The appearance of a foreign element and the chaos created by lack of boundaries finally pushed SFC to Rebellion, the next stage in its development as a therapeutic community.

3

Rebellion

After eight years as the leader of SFC, Virginia decided in 1984 to end her direct involvement in the camp. She made her announcement in a letter:

> July 10, 1984
> Dear Satir Family Camp Friends,
>
> It seems obvious to me after the last eight years experience that Family Camp offers a wealth of opportunities for enhancing, appreciating, and enjoying family life. Now that it is time for me to move on, the Satir Family Camp Committee has clearly embodied the values of healthy, physical, emotional and social family life. I feel certain that this committee is capable of sustaining and deepening and widening the fine foundation that has been built. Your participation will support this very important aim.
>
> When I started Family Camp eight years ago, I dreamed about the time when others would carry on this rewarding work. That time has come, and the committee is ready. With your help it will go far. I could not go unless I believed that were true.
>
> Lovingly,
> Virginia

Virginia's decision did not come as a complete surprise to the camp community. By the early 1980s, she was spending most of her time on international work. She traveled widely and presented trainings throughout the world. Particularly active in developing nations, she planned to use her skills and knowledge to help those countries address mental health issues. All who knew her saw that Virginia was determined to take her vision of healthy families and communities to the next level: helping create healthy states and nations.

Virginia also knew that sfc would become a stronger self-sustaining community when it was less dependent on her leadership. She did not withdraw completely, however. Even when leaving, she helped decide who would succeed her as the camp therapist. She knew it would be difficult for one person to inherit her role and so recommended that the Committee appoint a triad of therapists. Virginia was a strong advocate of using triads as a model for helping people learn and grow (Satir & Baldwin, 1983, pp. 171–75, 236). She also recommended using existing campers as the three therapists.

After each camp, Virginia met with members of the Committee to provide consultation. "This was a mutual need," reports a Committee member:

> Virginia certainly wanted to be involved, but it was our need as well. It was just so hard to let go of her presence and her input. It was almost like an annual pilgrimage to visit our guru. After each camp ended, members of the Committee drove up to Palo Alto and met with Virginia at her home. I think it really helped in the transition and probably would have gone on for a long while if she had not died.

Tragically, in 1988, Virginia's life was cut short after a brief struggle with pancreatic cancer. Although her death was a great personal loss to many campers, sfc continued to grow and thrive, just as Virginia had intended.

Transition: Therapy Program

After Virginia's resignation, the first challenge facing sfc's leaders was how to restructure the camp's therapeutic program now that it could no longer depend directly on Virginia's skill and leadership. As one Committee member said:

> Virginia was really wedded to this concept of the "triad." She used to have us do exercises in triads, and she felt that all leadership should be in triads. I guess the idea was that the triad was the original structure of Mother, Father, and Child. Well, at camp it didn't work all that well, particularly when the people she hand picked to be the first triad were just not that good.

A long-time camper held a similar view:

> I don't know if anyone could have succeeded as the therapist
> who followed Virginia. The measuring stick we used for the
> replacements was Virginia, of course, and there was no way anyone
> could come close to being Virginia. Then there was the problem that
> the people Virginia recommended were campers. That is a hard
> transition to make, going from camper to therapist. It's not surprising
> we rejected the first team. We just could not accept those folks in that
> different role. Right from the start, it was a set-up.

Several years after Virginia left, the Committee decided it needed
to make decisions based on the group's current needs rather than solely
on Virginia's recommendations. Many members were ready to develop
a camp based on Virginia's principles rather than her personality. The
Committee's shift away from Virginia's dominance to an era of self-
governance is evident in minutes of their November 1986 meeting:

> We . . . entered into an extensive and positive discussion of
> facilitation [therapy] for 1987, taking seriously the recommendations
> of the 1986 campers on that subject, as well as our own observations.
> We noted that we have a very different perspective than previously, as
> we approach our third year without the overriding presence of
> Virginia Satir. There was a decided preference for having two leaders,
> rather than three, and there was a general consensus that one of the
> leaders should be a man.

Camp moved from Rebellion to Redefinition somewhat seam-
lessly during the transition years. The energy of the Integration stage
of the Satir Change Model fueled the process of integrating the community's new ideas, resources, and expectations. In the transition's
first few years, pressure built in the group to return to the relative
comfort of earlier years under Virginia's powerful presence. The community made a series of trial-and-error attempts to redefine the structure, leadership roles, and program descriptions. Eventually, they
settled on elements of organization that continue today.

By the fourth year without Virginia, SFC had regained a sense of
balance and stability. The group became comfortable with a team of two
new facilitators, led by Laura Dodson. Laura first came to SFC as a camper
with her two children. She was Virginia's colleague, but as a parent of
young children, she easily connected with the young families, particularly

when she took the initiative to establish the Children's Program. After she presented a workshop on dreams at a Free University, the Committee asked her to become one of the therapists.

Although Laura had been a camper, her expertise as a therapist and the fact that the Committee recruited her for the job made it easier for the camp to accept her in the role of therapist. To this day, Laura continues to be the steering grace behind sfc's therapeutic program.

Transition: Community Governance

Choosing the camp's therapeutic leadership was a major first step in the Committee's assuming responsibility for all aspects of camp governance. Committee meetings evolved from discussing logistics and camp activities to addressing significant organizational issues. By 1988, the group had an Executive Committee, made up of the registrar and two others as well as a secretary. At its March 1988 meeting, Committee members identified what they wanted in a governance body (sfc Committee meeting minutes):

> . . . we wish the Committee to:
>
> Be inclusive
> Have continuity of membership
> Have a thoughtful commitment from those who wish to be on
>   the Committee
> Have members who have attended camp at least several years
> Have members who will attend all meetings
> Hold open meetings and have campers attend as observers

At that same meeting, the Committee discussed the "rock incident" (described in Chapter 2), focusing on how and if the Committee could or should manage campers' behavior. In part, the minutes read (1988, p. 4):

> . . . we agreed that the Committee or even the Executive
> Committee has the right and responsibility to ask any individual to
> leave camp immediately whose behavior jeopardizes the spirit of the
> camp and violates the values which we hold. [Committee members]
> will be prepared to do that, should the need arise.

In May 1988, the Committee reexamined this statement and discussed it further. This deeper discussion and reaction are hallmarks of how the Committee uses process both to discuss issues and make decisions. That meeting's minutes report:

> . . . When the discussion and conclusion [excerpted above] were synopsized and reported on paper in black and white, they had a different impact than when the issue was dynamically discussed, in a larger context . . . [about] the function of the Committee and its Executive Committee. . . .
>
> . . . sitting in the trees in Big Sur [the May meeting's location], the Committee realized that we had arrived at a conclusion without clearly setting down the process through which that conclusion was arrived. We had a lengthy, difficult, and sometimes painful discussion of the values of sfc, the ways we live and work together, in camp and out, the role of the Committee, and the functioning of the Executive Committee.
>
> We agreed that we had all assumed the content of our sessions at Pico Blanco would be regarded as confidential, and we realized that requirement has not been explicitly expressed in the past, but it shall be in the future. We have realized that some of us have had grievances against each other which we have not handled properly; they have been discussed with others, and sometimes never discussed with the party in question. We informally committed ourselves to be more faithful to each other and our values in the future.
>
> We acknowledged the responsibility for the operations, maintenance, and future of sfc and its values rests with the Committee, and we renewed our commitment to exercise those responsibilities thoughtfully and effectively. We will call upon the sfc therapists to consult with the Committee about the way we manage our responsibilities and to use that information educationally with the larger membership.

The Committee had thus evolved from an ad hoc group providing logistical support to Virginia and the landowners, into a group of volunteers who accepted responsibility for the camp and its operation. In a significant reversal of roles, the Committee became the primary decision maker while the therapist(s) and landowners assumed a supportive role.

At the May 1988 meeting, the Committee further established both the structure and the process for sfc governance. It also addressed key issues that the organization continues to struggle with almost twenty years later. These issues include: confidentiality of the work sessions; how campers relate to each other, especially when they disagree; and the roles and responsibilities of the Committee and the Executive Committee.

Although frustrating to some members who would prefer to focus on decisions and reach closure, this process of discussion and re-discussion is a living example of Virginia Satir's principles. Even when a decision is made, it may not always be the correct decision. Consensus decision making means that any decision can and should be re-visited and re-discussed when any member has a concern. Though frustrating and cumbersome, governance that uses group process and decision by consensus has helped sfc grow as both a community and an organization. This type of governance exists in stark contrast to the authoritarian control that Virginia exerted as leader. Again, the sfc overcame Virginia's personal limitations to live out her professional beliefs. At the 1990 camp, the Committee worked in front of the whole community to demonstrate its decision-making process and to improve their work together as a process group.

In 1991, sfc was thriving. Laura Dodson continued as the primary therapist. She had assumed a comfortable working relationship with the Committee and had the confidence and support of the general camp. Because the previous male co-therapist could not continue, Laura recruited Tom and Maureen Graves. Trained as Satir therapists, they attended in 1991 as campers, planning to begin as therapists in 1992.

By 1991, the camp had a strong Children's Program as well as an ongoing teen group to meet the needs of its ever-increasing adolescent population. Issues existed regarding late arrivals, integrating new members, concern about diversity, struggles with gossip, and confidentiality; but in general, the sfc felt secure and comfortable with its transition from Virginia's leadership to self-governance. And then the rains came.

The Accident

On Friday, July 1, the 1991 camp was coming to a close after a week of on-and-off rain. As campers endured yet another wet breakfast, the usual light rain turned torrential. Campers began to worry about the road over the mountain, wondering if it would become impassable due to the mud. Campers who were there that day provided the following descriptions. We have changed people's names to maintain confidentiality.

> There was kind of this feeling of free-floating anxiety in the camp. There was more than just the rain that people were worried about. There had been an earthquake in Southern California, and people from that area were particularly anxious to get home. It wasn't a big earthquake but it added to people's anxiety.

While the campers huddled under the blue tarps spread over the kitchen, the members of the Committee, along with the therapist and landowner, gathered to discuss options. If people were to leave, it needed to happen quickly. Another option was to wait until the rain stopped, but the concern remained that even without the rain the road could still be impassable. Worries were also expressed about how much food was available and if it could be kept safe for consumption. Despite some people on the Committee wanting to wait out the rains, the decision was made to leave camp that day. [See photo 9 in the section just before Part Two.]

As the announcement spread through camp, there were mixed reactions. Many campers were relieved. They were wet, cold, and more than ready to go home. Others were upset about ending camp with no process or closure. Still others felt anxious about going over the mountain and wanted to wait until the rain stopped. This decision was not open to group process, however, and the evacuation commenced immediately. Campsites were dismantled and groups of families hiked up the road to Harry's trailer where the trucks and some Committee members' cars were parked. From there, groups were to be driven up and over the top of the mountain to the camp's larger parking lot.

> As we look back, it is easy to say it wasn't the best decision to make and certainly the process didn't work well. Clearly, we did not think through the risks. We all just kind of accepted that Harry would get us out like he always did.
> Not all of us agreed with the decision. We did all go up to Harry's trailer and most people left, but I was not willing to risk my family on that road. We spent the night at the trailer and by the next day, the sun came out and the road was passable.

Wilson, who did decide to leave, described the events with a detachment that belies the dire consequences his family faced that fateful day.

> We had a long way to drive after we got out of camp, so I wanted to get all of us out as quickly as possible. We were among the first group to get to Harry's trailer. Our car was parked there, so my sons—Keenan and Danny—and I got in the car while my wife, Eva, and daughter, Kirsten, followed behind us on the first camp truck. When I got in the car, I thought about how I had felt when I drove into camp. On the ride down, I had said to Eva, "Sometimes I feel I'm just going over the edge." That statement came back to me as we began to drive out. I'd come to camp

pretty depressed, had not really gotten much out of camp that week, and here we were, having to drive out in a sea of mud, heading for disaster.

Kirsten, then 14, also remembered leaving camp with a sense of foreboding:

> At the start of the day, when it was decided that we would evacuate, I had a bad gut feeling about it. But, it was one of those things that you just hush inside of you and proceed because it was something that needed to be done. I can remember being worried as I watched my dad and brothers start their hike up to the car.

When Wilson and the boys got into the car, Wilson had a sense that things might not go smoothly.

> I remember telling the kids not to put on seat belts "in case we have to jump out" so I guess I sort of knew we might have problems. As we were going down the hill, we got to this curve where the embankment was on the inside and it was just a cliff on the outside. I remember I tried to avoid the edge as we made the turn and then all of a sudden, I knew we were going over. The car started to slide and I yelled, "This is it!" and we were flying, and then I woke up on the ground.

As Wilson and the boys drove into the curve, Eva and Kirsten were behind them, unaware of what was happening. Kirsten describes how they became aware that Wilson and the boys were gone.

> My mom and I, along with other campers, loaded into the back of a camp truck and started down the hill. The ride was very scary, slipping and sliding, and some campers chose to get out and walk. I stayed in the truck, trusting Harry and his knowledge of the roads and the land. The next thing I remember is seeing tire tracks. Harry drove right on them, even as we were all yelling that something was wrong. He finally stopped and as I jumped out of the truck, I ran over to the cliff and at some point I saw my brother Keenan. He was covered in blood. That's when I started screaming.

Eva recalled the horror of that moment.

> I remember everyone yelling about an accident. I think it was Raymond [another camper] who kept hitting the cab of the truck and telling Harry to stop. Then I heard Kirsten screaming, "No Mommy, no, Mommy!" I knew it was Wilson who had gone over, and I was sure Kirsten was looking at dead bodies.

Wilson continued:

> Danny and I were both thrown out, but Keenan went down with
> the car. I remember hearing Danny crying out over and over, "I love
> you, Daddy. I love you, Daddy." I tried to get up to find him, and
> that's when I knew something was really wrong. I was just pinned
> and couldn't move. Then I could hear Keenan yelling. I didn't know
> where either of them was. I could just hear their voices, and I guess
> they could hear mine.

It turned out that Keenan was the least hurt. Although lucky not
to be ejected from the car, he had been thrown into the back seat, and
the car ended up landing in a tree. Wilson remembered:

> Somehow he got out of the car, which was jammed up in a tree,
> about six to eight feet off the ground, and started climbing up the hill.
> I told him, "Find Danny. Find Danny." I think what he did was climb
> up to the road to get help.

At this point, help first arrived. Raymond and his wife Melissa,
both physicians, were on the truck with Eva and Kirsten. Raymond
commented:

> We were all fortunate that we had resources within camp to
> provide some medical care, as we were a long way from any hospital.
> Melissa and I were able to assess things, but it was really Devina
> [another camper who was an emergency room doctor and got to the
> scene shortly after Raymond and Melissa] who took charge of the site
> and cared for Wilson.

While Melissa helped to assess and care for Danny and Keenan
alongside the road, Raymond went to the crash site. He described
what he found:

> I can't believe they survived. The car was just jammed in the
> branches of a tree over six feet off the ground. The engine had been
> forced into the front seat. No one would have lived if they had had
> their seat belts on. Of course, it was a miracle that they survived
> being thrown out, as well. Wilson was caught on a branch, which
> caused most of his injuries but also probably saved his life. Keenan
> made it because he was thrown into the back with all the camping
> gear that kind of cushioned him when the car landed in the tree. It's
> amazing . . . both Keenan and Danny actually walked out. They had a
> lot of cuts and bruises but their biggest complaint afterward was about

the poison oak they got when climbing to the road! Wilson, on the other hand, was seriously injured, and it was touch and go getting him out of there. He's lucky he has not only his life but his leg as well.

Wilson has only hazy recollections of the time before he was rescued.

> They tell me I was on the hillside for about five hours. I kind of went in and out. I remember hearing the emergency guys talking about how big I was and what it would take to get me out of there. For a long time, they didn't give me anything for the pain. Finally, Raymond took responsibility for the pain medication, and they gave me a shot. If Raymond hadn't been there, they wouldn't have given me anything because they were out of radio contact with the hospital. Good thing he was, 'cause eventually they had to use a winch to get me off the hillside.

Wilson had major injuries and the boys, although not physically injured in a major way, were badly traumatized. The following is Danny's description of the accident, which occurred when he was ten years old.

> I remember the car going over like it was kind of slow motion. If Dad hadn't told us to not wear seat belts, we probably would have all died. I remember him opening the door to jump out, I guess, and then all I remember is screaming, "I love you, Daddy. I love you, Daddy."
>
> Then I was on the ground. Later on, Keenan just showed up. He was all covered in blood, which kind of freaked me out, but I guess he was okay 'cause he got up to the top first and got help. I climbed up after him.
>
> What I remember most about being hurt is having poison oak. I had the worst case of poison oak I ever had before or since. I guess we got it when we crawled up the hillside.

In the meantime, Kirsten and Eva were forced to wait at the side of the road as the boys crawled up and Wilson remained hidden from sight. Kirsten continued the story:

> It turned out that Keenan only suffered minor cuts and bruises but, unaware of that, all I could see was blood, and it really scared me. Danny was able to get up to the top of the cliff, too, and I knew he was okay. Soon after that, I could hear my dad talking but I didn't see

him. He was down a way and couldn't move. I think I saw him once during the rescue efforts.

Once the boys reached the road, Eva faced the choice all mothers dread when more than one member of their family needs support during a trauma:

It was the hardest choice I ever made, but I decided to stay with Wilson until they got him evacuated. I knew he had the greatest need right then, but I also wanted to be with the boys, and there was Kirsten as well. But in the end it was the right place to be. He was in so much pain and they took so long to decide whether they could give him some medicine. And I knew that the kids would be okay because they were with family . . . the Satir Family Camp family.

Kirsten described how she coped after her mother went to help her dad.

My mom stayed with him while I calmed down and stayed with my little brother Danny. He was lying to the side of the road with a hurt leg. I can remember as the rest of the cars drove by to evacuate camp, it was terrifying to me. Our car had been a big four-wheel-drive Suburban, and other people were trying to get out in little tiny cars. I watched them slide around, as they zig-zagged around with no traction.

I was afraid of something happening to someone else; and even more, I was very afraid that someone would catch the same slide that my dad had and get shot down the cliff and roll over the people helping or over my dad stuck on the hill. I remember being very scared about any of us getting into a car to get the rest of the way down the hill, including my brothers' being in the ambulance.

Danny described the challenge of his final evacuation to the hospital:

After I got to the top, I had to be driven down to an ambulance. I was put into a car with this cop who started driving and really freaked me out. He kept saying over and over, "Oh god, we're sliding." That sure didn't make me feel great, but when we got to the ambulance, they put me in with Keenan, and I felt a little better. The hospital was really hard. They took Keenan and me in together, but then they put me in a room by myself and just kind of left me there. It seemed like forever and no one came to see about me. I didn't know where my mom was. I figured she needed to be with my dad. But they wouldn't let me be with Keenan or anyone. Finally, I saw my dad go by on the stretcher. And then I heard him scream this just *awful* scream, and I really lost it and started screaming myself.

Kirsten had the same memory of Wilson's arrival and treatment in the emergency room:

> I can't remember who I left with or how I got to the emergency room. I do remember that at the hospital, I was in the waiting room and I heard my dad screaming louder than I'd ever heard anyone screaming. I think he screamed until he passed out from the pain.

At that point, Eva moved all three children to the care of SFC campers. Danny remembered:

> After I lost it, mom came in and they got me in a wheelchair and let me go out in the waiting room. And all of Family Camp was there. I can't tell you how great that felt. It was like the whole camp was there to care for me.

One of the Committee members described the Family Camp response.

> That hospital did not know what hit them. There we all were, most of us covered in mud and just tracking it all over that E.R. We all got hotel rooms in Monterey, and we just stayed there to care for the kids and be a support to Eva and 'cause we couldn't leave until we knew Wilson was okay.

Leaving Pico Blanco

Although severely shaken by the accident, the Committee remained committed to continuing camp at Pico Blanco. Wilson and his family slowly recovered from their injuries and trauma. At its November meeting, the Committee addressed the accident and its impact on the campers as well as the organization. The minutes of the meeting reflect both individual and community responses (SFC Committee Meeting minutes, November 9–10, 1991).

> There was a special energy in the air as we gathered for the first time following our emergency departure from the mud of Bug Sur six weeks earlier. Many of us had last seen each other at the Monterey Peninsula Hospital where we visited with Wilson and Eva and the children immediately following their disastrous crash. It was a relief to see Wilson, holding court in a large armchair, crutches by his side, with a broad smile on his face.

For two hours before lunch, we relived the complex moments preceding our evacuation, during the evacuation, and following our departure from camp. Many tears were shed. We sat holding hands, locking arms, listening intently to hear how it was for our friends. A completed picture emerged when twenty different perspectives were shared. A more adequate closure was reached.

The remainder of that meeting focused on the risks involved in holding a residential camp for over eighty people in a wilderness environment. The Committee reviewed emergency procedures and discussed legal implications for the camp as a whole and for the Committee as its governing body. The minutes indicate the Committee's growing awareness of the camp's need for a more formal organization (SFC Committee meeting, November 9–10, 1991).

> We recognized that it has become necessary to provide liability insurance for the entire camp, as well as for the Committee. We confronted ourselves with the ugly truth that the accident victims of June 1991 could sue the Executive Committee, the full Committee, and every person at camp, as well as the landowners. Further we need specifically to obtain insurance for the Board Members. So, after all these years, we decided to incorporate, apply for tax-exempt status, and cover ourselves with insurance.

Until then, the Committee had functioned without a legal structure. Now, it to once again expanded its role and responsibilities.

During this meeting, the Committee discussed the letter sent to the camp by the owners of the Pico Blanco land. The letter listed conditions that SFC would have to meet if it continued to camp at Pico Blanco. The Committee reviewed the list and decided to have the Executive Committee meet with the owners to see if any compromise could be reached.

Although the Executive Committee had that meeting and discussed all the options, they could not achieve a compromise. The proposed restrictions increased SFC's financial burden and made it unfeasible to continue using the Pico Blanco site. The Committee also decided that camping in an isolated area prone both to rain and wildfires posed too great a risk for SFC families. Within four months, they selected a new location, SFC became incorporated, and the Camp Loma years began.

Community Implications

During the transition years following Virginia's departure and through the move to Camp Loma, the community concentrated more on boundaries. The *Lord of the Flies* incident and the snake incident pushed the community toward developing greater structure and defining more boundaries. This led to the stage of Redefinition, the community focused its energy on integrating the new structure. It is the energy of Integration that fuels both the developmental stage of Redefinition and the transition years of the camp.

As campers noted in their descriptions, Virginia's presence had always seemed enough to handle any and all crises. Her undisputed leadership steered the course through obstacles and the Definition and Establishment stages of the community's growth. With her absence, leadership sometimes wavered, and the course for the community was not always clear. While the Committee took steps to define their roles and responsibilities, the community continued the process of separation and independence necessary in development.

The first signs of the community's assertion for independence came with its departure from the leadership triad endorsed by Virginia as well as its development of the Children's Program to impose structure and supervision on the children's time at camp. These aspects of the community were redefined in the transition period.

Committee minutes suggest some evidence of Virginia's internal conflict around the community's independence. Virginia emphasized her ideas for leadership even when the community felt the triad of therapists was not working for sfc. However, she gradually moved away from her involvement in camp until she had completely left the community to its own designs and development. She seemed to recognize that her continued leadership and active role in the camp/community would hamper the next stages of development. As parents have done for all time, she pushed the childlike community to stand on its own and find its own sense of independence and self-confidence.

After the accident, the camp cycled back into the Rebellion stage. Camp had been operating in the Establishment stage in which the defined structure had been meeting the needs of the majority of camp. However, the rains presented a new and dangerous energy of the Foreign Element to consider. With the subsequent accident came campers' strong emotional reactions and a significant challenge to how camp had operated up to then.

The Satir Theory of Change sees the campers' fears and concerns as the fuel of the Chaos stage. The energies of the Foreign Element and of Chaos reactivated the stage of Rebellion. Throughout the year following the accident, campers expressed concerns about a variety of issues. They worried about the safety of the Pico Blanco location, and the landowners worried about their liability. Campers challenged how the decision to evacuate was made and second-guessed the camp leaders. This close scrutiny was a function of the stage of Rebellion.

4

Redefinition

Once the camp moved to Camp Loma, the community faced more changes. Stimulating these changes were a shift in the power structure as well as a drastic decrease in the isolation that had been Pico Blanco. In 2004, a camper described Camp Loma:

> When I arrive at Camp Loma early Friday, I am struck by how old and tattered it appears. There is a vast field of dry grass and dirt surrounding a covered concrete dining area that is filled with decrepit picnic tables and benches, as well as dirt, and pine cones. The majestic redwoods that fill the campgrounds seem empty and forlorn. The magic that is Satir Family Camp has yet to arrive. Slowly during the day, carefully driven autos enter the meadow to disgorge their contents onto the barren field. A small group of about twenty families quickly spread into the woods surrounding the camp buildings. These are members of the Committee who have arrived a day early to set up the physical camp, which has sat unused since the previous summer. Here and there a green or yellow tent billows up. Paths up the hillsides are reestablished as more and more supplies are carried up and vanish into the tents that spread color among the trees. Voices begin to filter into the air.
> The latrines are unlocked and swept clean. The kitchen is opened, scrubbed of cobwebs and dirt and filled with food and supplies. The old and scarred picnic tables are disbursed onto the grounds, covered with green table cloths, and crowned with a cheerful plant or cup of flowers. "The Bin," a large storage container where much of the sfc supplies are kept during the year, is slowly emptied. Camping equipment, an unending supply of camping chairs, the Session area baffles [large pieces of wood covered with fabric to

facilitate sound], the latrine supplies, the children's program supplies, and detritus from almost twenty-five years of camping is sent out into the camp. The Bin is then replenished with boxes of paper towels, toilet paper, and nonperishable foods that will be used during the upcoming week.

Folding tables that will hold the ever abundant amounts of food are set up for the more meager provisions made by the Committee for themselves. Peanut butter and jelly, bread and bagels, fruit and more fruit is put out to nourish those who labor to get camp ready for opening at mid day on Saturday. As the work is finished for the day, a fire is set in the fire pit, chairs are put out around it, and the first night of pre-camp comes to a close with old friends catching up on current events or reminiscing about the dramas of camps gone by.

Arrival Day

The day begins with a Committee meeting to review final assignments. Airport pickups are arranged, volunteers are assigned to the welcoming committee, and new camper mentors are recruited. The inevitable last-minute crises rear their ugly heads. There is a lack of power in one of the latrines. Do we have enough water pressure? Oh god, someone plugged a toilet *already*!

Through it all, the energy builds towards 2 p.m. when the larger contingent of campers begins to arrive. Hoots and hollers float in the air as old campers return and new families are greeted with enthusiasm. Cars wait in line to park in the few areas around camp where it is safe to unpack. Tents, backpacks, duffel bags and, here and there, a suitcase are unloaded and hauled up the hillsides to remote or close-by camping areas. The wires strung around the kitchen and dining area suddenly sprout a variety of plastic bags holding each family's dining ware. The children's area becomes a beehive of activity. Supplies are unpacked and organized into drawers and onto shelves while children wander through, looking at games and projects they can work on during the week. The volleyball net is set up, ping pong games begin, but mostly the arrival activities consist of hugs and lots and lots of talking among friends, many of whom have not seen each other for a year.

This very old and worn 4H Camp has again, for this one week, become a Family Camp. Amidst laughter and sometimes a few tears, friends and awkward new arrivals mix and anticipate the week ahead. For me, as I look out from my campsite over the quiet hillside that had been empty just the night before, the Magical Village has arisen yet again. It brings back memories of playing with a toy village I had been given one Christmas. My fantasy village is created before me, full of real people who come together for one week a year to live in the magic known as Satir Family Camp.

When sᴆ held its first camp at Camp Loma in 1992, two Committee members had less prosaic reactions:

> Probably the biggest difference between Camp Loma and Pico Blanco is Camp Loma's accessibility. You drive up in your car, get out and unload, and you are there. No packing up to get onto the trucks, no crazy ride down the mountain, and saddest of all, no sense of us being totally alone in the world.
>
> It was so hard to leave Pico Blanco. Yes, we knew it was dangerous and that we were lucky not to have lost Wilson and the boys or to have anyone else injured. But Pico Blanco was Satir Family Camp. That was the place where we grew up and of course that is where Virginia was with us. But in the end I think we all knew that camp is more than a place and we were just so grateful to be able to have camp meet again that the place became less important. And now I really appreciate the conveniences.

Camp Loma, owned by the Santa Cruz Youth Agency and used primarily as a campsite for 4Her's, was an attractive option for many who had not been happy with the isolation of Pico Blanco. For some campers, the only reason they returned to sᴆ was because the camp was accessible and easily evacuated.

Tess Returns

As she promised herself, Tess did not return to sᴆ for many years. She did, however, maintain her friendship with Alicia. Although they had an agreement not to discuss Tess's return to sᴆ, Alicia managed to share some interesting or funny story after each year's camp. Despite her personal fears, Tess found herself interested in the stories. The farther away she got from her personal experience at camp, the more she let herself become aware of how the one week she spent at sᴆ helped her better understand her inner experiences and their effect on her daily life.

When Alicia came back from camp in 1991 and told her about the horror of the evacuation and the accident, Tess's feelings were mixed. On the one hand, the accident reinforced her belief that she had been lucky to survive her week at sᴆ. On the other hand, she shared Alicia's grief that this might be the end of camp.

Tess found she was actually pleased to hear that sᴆ had found a new location and that it would continue. She described how her reconnection came about.

In the back of my mind, I knew sfc was very special and I really did want it to be there in case I ever felt I could return. It just happened that the first year they held sfc at Camp Loma, Alicia needed a ride home. I had planned a vacation in the area for that week and agreed to pick her up when camp was over on Saturday.

When Tess drove up to Camp Loma, she was struck by the difference in the camp.

The campers' cars were parked right there at the camp. There was a whole parking lot of cars by this road, an actual paved road that ran right through the middle of camp. The road took you into the campsite and then took you right back down the mountain. When I drove there, I realized it took only about 30 minutes to get from this camp to a town, and I thought, "This place is really safe." Then, when Alicia showed me around, I was so impressed by the luxury of the accommodations—well, luxurious compared to Pico Blanco, of course. This camp had bathrooms and showers in real buildings and segregated by sex. Even the individual showers had shower curtains so you could have a totally private shower!

And while we were walking through the camp, people kept coming up to me and they remembered my name and of course had to have a hug, which actually felt pretty good. A lot of them asked me when I was coming back. I began to have this glimmer of awareness that these people were really seeing me, Tess. It felt genuine and it felt good. When Alicia and I drove back down the coast, we did a lot of talking and I realized not only do I think I can go there but I want to go back.

The following year, Tess returned to camp and has been attending ever since.

Camp Loma Campsite

Camp Loma does not offer luxury accommodations, but a number of its conveniences have balanced some of the sense of loss many original campers felt after leaving Pico Blanco. An Olympic-size swimming pool provides enjoyment for adults and children, as long as they can tolerate unheated and often bone-chilling water. The latrines and showers are in buildings that provide a sense of privacy. The well-worn kitchen is in a building and includes a walk-in cooler, several large freezers, two restaurant-size ranges with ovens, and four large sinks for preparing food and washing dishes. The covered eating area provides a sheltered place for meetings as well as eating and a sink for campers to wash their dishes. [See photos 10–16 in the section just before Part Two.]

The major drawback for those who came from Pico Blanco was the road. It provides access to the camp but also divides the camp-ground. Most of the main activities in camp occur in the "lower area" on the road's south side. This area has the kitchen, dining area, fire pit, amphitheater, Children's Program corner, teen room, recreation field, pool, showers and bathrooms (attached to the pool), a playing field, and an area for the work sessions. The surrounding hillsides are used for camping.

The "upper area" on the road's north side includes another set of showers and toilets, the parking area, and hillside space that is used only for camping. From the beginning, sfc requested that all families with children under age 8 camp in the lower area to minimize the need for these children to cross the road. Despite initial concerns about safety, sfc children and the community as a whole have adjusted well to the openness of the Camp Loma site.

Change Factors

The Camp Loma phase of sfc began in 1992. In addition to being the first sfc to be held at Camp Loma, other forces came together to make 1992 a year of breakthroughs and changes.

Accepting a New Campsite

As much as campers had to deal with the physical changes in the move to Camp Loma, they also had to cope with symbolic changes it represented. They were no longer isolated in a magic wonderland that was theirs alone. Instead, they were using a facility shared by other groups who camped at the site after sfc. This lack of isolation led to a different sense in camp. Veteran campers described this change:

> We were no longer this special group living in our own world. There was a road rather than a creek in the middle of our community. We worried not only about the kids being safe but of our becoming divided between those camping on one side or the other of a road!

> As wonderful as it is to have a real kitchen and bathrooms that do not open to the sky, it begins to feel like a summer camp instead of Family Camp. I think there is a real risk that sfc has become just another summer vacation. That could never happen at Pico Blanco. There was just not anyone who would go to Pico Blanco for a vacation. You went there for Family Camp. Unfortunately, I don't think that is true at Camp Loma.

New Facilitators

As the previous chapter mentioned, Maureen and Tom Graves came to SFC as campers in 1991 and as therapists in 1992. Both had trained with Virginia and also had experience and expertise in the areas of drug and alcohol abuse and child sex abuse. Laura Dodson had observed that more people were raising these issues at camp, and she thought when she recruited them that Maureen and Tom could help her meet more of the camp's needs. With very little discussion, the Committee agreed to hire the Graves. As one Committee member said, "We knew that Laura would be traveling more and might not be as available to come to camp. We just wanted to be sure we would have facilitators every camp and were willing to accept Laura's recommendation."

Status of the Landowners

For the first time, the Pico Blanco landowners came to camp as campers without additional status. This was a significant shift both for them and for SFC. For some campers, the fact that SFC was now renting the facilities from an organization rather than from individuals was an important step toward making camp more democratic. For others, the owners of the Pico Blanco site remained the camp's guardian angels. As one long-time camper said:

> Without their efforts, as well as connections, there wouldn't have been any camp that year. They found Camp Loma for us and convinced the Santa Cruz Youth Agency to let a group of families who were not affiliated with the 4H organization camp there. I know some people resented their special status and all, but to me they . . . along with Virginia . . . really made SFC work.

Unfortunately, the change in their role, both for the owners and for the camp, was never bridged successfully, and they did not return as campers after 1992.

Old vs. New Campers

The change in location also resulted in a new difference among campers. The move created yet another subgroup: those who had never camped at Pico Blanco. Virginia's departure in 1984 had yielded a slight differentiation among campers who had attended when Virginia was present and those who came after she left. Somehow, this distinction did not seem very significant until the move to Camp Loma. It may not have been as important at Pico Blanco because in the years following Virginia's departure, new families came at a moderate rate. When sfc moved to Camp Loma, however, sfc deliberately recruited new families. They came to camp lacking not only direct experience with Virginia but also the shared history of being at Pico Blanco. It is likely that some of these new campers would not have chosen to camp in a location like Pico Blanco. This and other factors caused a shift in the culture of the camp as it settled into its new environment.

Increasing Isolation of the Adolescents

A teen group had started at Pico Blanco. Now, at Camp Loma, the Committee gave the group its own space to meet and to hang out. This eventually had consequences for the camp as a whole, as explained by a camper and former teen group facilitator:

> A lot of the issues involving the teens kind of came to a head after we moved to Camp Loma. When we got to Camp Loma, we decided to give them their own space and to really encourage them to bond together as a group. On the one hand, this let them play their music and be loud at night, which was great. But eventually we realized that the teens were hanging out only with each other and becoming more and more removed from the larger community. And as the teen group grew larger, some of their "exploratory" behavior became more obvious to the larger community.

Confronting the Status Quo

As Virginia discussed in her Change Theory Model, change creates and sometimes forces people to confront issues that have often remained hidden during periods of Status Quo. After the move, as one Committee member described:

> Everything was so different at Camp Loma. In some ways it was almost like starting a new camp. We had a lot of new people and of course new traditions had to be started. I don't think it's surprising that we also began to deal with some of our old issues in new ways.

A male camper said:

> It was a challenging camp that year. We had to deal with what had happened at the end of our time at Pico Blanco as well as the new

environment of Camp Loma. This was also the year that several women chose to deal with issues related to molestation, which creates a separate tension because that is such a painful issue for the individual to confront and for all of us who know and care for them to watch.

By the time sFc moved to Camp Loma, attitudes toward sexual issues, particularly childhood molestation, had changed dramatically. Initially, at Pico Blanco, most of the relationships between the sexes reflected the cultural attitudes of the 1960s and 1970s, particularly attitudes on the West Coast and within the human potential movement. It was common in that era for men and women to share showers and to participate in nude swimming and sunbathing. Activities at Pico Blanco—group showers, nude swimming and sunbathing, and sexual involvement among campers—reflected these attitudes. Some saw sexual intimacy as a natural extension of the emotional intimacy fostered at camp. Sexual contact occurred between and among married as well as single partners. Those campers who attended sFc during that period generally agree that sex was not the primary reason people went to camp. Rather, it was something that was just a part of camp in the same way that sex and open relationships were part of the broader culture. As the years passed and societal attitudes changed, most behaviors also changed at sFc. Unfortunately, not all campers made such changes. Concerns around sexual behavior in camp grew. By the time sFc moved to Camp Loma, those concerns had grown into unspoken tension. As a male camper put it, "I think having new facilitators, a new place, and, for us, a lot of new people who did not have old relationships just set the stage for what happened."

The Elephant in the Room

What happened that year was a major confrontation between the community and two campers who, in the opinion of many women, had been inappropriate in their sexual behavior. After interviewing campers who were present when the confrontation occurred, we wrote the following story, changing the names of campers and approximating their conversations.

Within a few years of camp beginning at Pico Blanco, Mick's sexual behavior became an issue for some campers. Although people talked about it informally, particularly the female campers, it was years before the sFc community actually addressed the issue with

Mick, in what this book calls "the Mick Incident." Looking back on the events that led to that, most campers agree that Virginia had to leave camp, the camp itself had to leave Pico Blanco, and the Committee had to step into a leadership role before the community could confront Mick about his inappropriate sexual advances.

Much of the campers' reluctance to confront the issue was tied to the fact that Mick and his wife Rose enjoyed a privileged status at camp. Many campers perceived them as having power, some acknowledged but most unspoken, at SFC. They had attended the pre–Pico Blanco camp and were major contributors to the planning for camp. They also donated both time and money to help pay for the use of land, both at Pico Blanco and initially at Camp Loma. While Virginia was at SFC, Mick and Rose were part of her Inner Circle. They camped next to Virginia and took part in the visits to Harry's trailer.

Initially, Mick sought out sexual contacts during camp in the same manner as other men in camp. These men enjoyed looking at and appreciating women. If the women were agreeable, sexual activity could and did occur. As some of the original campers look back on that period, they are uncertain when Mick's behavior changed from a search for sexual liaisons to, in today's terminology, "inappropriate" behavior. It was always clear that Mick enjoyed women and that he considered himself attractive to them. He was not shy about sharing his enjoyment of sex with the women at camp. He considered camp a time to "let down your hair and be who you are," and for Mick that was being a connoisseur of women. He enjoyed watching girls blossom into womanhood and he felt privileged to share his appreciation with them.

At first, Mick's unwelcome sexual behavior was mostly verbal. He never hesitated to comment on the loveliness of the ladies at camp in a manner that on the surface was not offensive, but he delivered these remarks in a tone and with nonverbal expressions that some women found uncomfortable. Gradually, he began to take advantage of the famous camp hugs. He used the friendly hug as a way to partake in the delights of a young as well as a mature woman's body. Women campers dealt with Mick's behavior in a variety of ways:

> All the women knew you had to watch his hands and whenever possible avoid him when he wanted to hug.

> The first year I came to camp, I became friendly with Suzanne. As we were talking about different campers and who was who, she said, very casually, "Oh, by the way, watch out for Mick's hands."

I asked her, "What do you mean?"

"Oh you know," she told me, "he's just one of those guys who thinks he's god's gift to women. Just remember, he will try to take advantage if you give him an opening."

From then on, I made sure I never got near enough to Mick to really find out what she meant. It's funny, now that I think about it, part of me always kind of wondered if he just didn't find me attractive! Kind of shows you how much women were indoctrinated in those days. And he was part of the "in group," so part of me felt a little left out when he ignored me. I think that was some of the reason so many people put up with it. Kind of like if Mick paid attention to you, then you were part of the "in group." But when he was finally confronted and I heard how angry everyone was, I guess I'm really glad I never got on his radar.

A camper who had been an adolescent girl during this time at Pico Blanco reported:

It was his lecherous looks that really made me sick. The worst part was when you were in the showers. See, most of us were just developing, and to have him there looking us over was gross. I just never showered if Mick was around, and if he came in when I was showering, I always left.

Despite his known behaviors and the developing negative reaction to them, no one spoke up directly to Mick, the Committee, or Virginia. Instead, the women looked out for each other. They developed ways to let each other know if Mick was heading toward the showers. If one woman was caught in a "Mick hug," another woman would quickly approach and begin talking to interrupt the process. "And in the end, if it happened, you grinned and bore it and got away as quickly as you could," said one of the women from the young families.

For the men, it was more frustrating. In the end, most of them viewed Mick as kind of pathetic. Nelson stated:

I knew Phyllis could take care of herself. We did talk about it, but mostly to make a joke and kind of feel sorry for him. We felt a lot sorrier for Rose because we really liked her and felt that Mick's behavior kind of humiliated her.

One time, though, I really lost all respect and tolerance for Mick. We had had a men's group and I had shared some feelings regarding Phyllis that were not only personal but confidential to that group. Later in the evening I learned, from Phyllis no less, that Mick had gone to her and shared what I had said. It was difficult enough to know that Mick had violated the group confidentiality. But what really got me was that he used the information almost like a come-on with Phyllis. After that, I was done with any respect I had for Mick, and it sure affected how I felt when the storm finally hit.

The "storm" occurred soon after the move to Camp Loma. The entire week had been challenging. People were still adjusting to the new site, and the community as a whole seemed less cohesive and a bit out of sorts. The therapeutic work had focused on sexual issues, particularly child molestation, and many campers felt quite vulnerable. Eliana, Nita, and Marx were relatively new as a therapy team and, unexpectedly, Eliana had to leave camp a day early. That left Nita and Marx responsible for ending the therapeutic sessions at camp. At first, much of the energy that became the "elephant in the room" focused on one new family. From the moment Pierre and Pauline arrived, it was obvious that they were "different." As one long-term camper said,

> I know judging by outer appearances isn't fair, but I'll tell you in this case it was pretty clear just by their appearance that Pierre and Pauline were different from most of us at camp. The way they looked and spoke, they just kind of stood out. Pauline always looked to me like she was going square dancing. The first day I saw her, I thought maybe she thought it was Party Night. Now I can understand that on the first day, she may have thought that was a great outfit. But you know, once you get a sense that your dress is a bit out of the ordinary, I guess I kind of assume you would change. I mean, lord knows we don't have a dress code at camp, but most of us are dressed for camping. Standing out like that just never seemed to make a bit of difference to them, though!

Had the issues been simply outer appearances, the community may have isolated the family a bit, but it is unlikely people would have remained concerned. Campers often see many families as kind of unusual the first year they come to camp. Returning campers often wonder if the new families "really fit in." Yet, after several summers, as the new campers relax and share, particularly at work sessions, long-time campers accept many of those they saw initially as peculiar or unorthodox. The newcomers become valuable members of the community.

Unfortunately, events unfolded very differently for Pierre and Pauline due mostly to Pierre's sexual proclivities. By the end of the week, rumors spread through camp that Pierre was photographing women in the showers and hiding in the bushes to spy on women as they dressed in their campsites. This behavior did bring formal complaints to the Committee by several adolescent women who were unwilling to have the matter "just talked about." These young women "wanted something done about him."

The Executive Committee discussed the issue with the therapists and struggled over how to deal with the complaints while supporting Pierre and his family. During the Executive Committee's discussion, it came to light that at least one of the reports of Pierre photographing women from the bushes was inaccurate. In fact, a female camper had requested that Pierre photograph her. This contradictory information created additional concern regarding not only how to approach the issue but how accurate the issue was in the first place.

As more people in camp spoke among themselves and more women expressed their discomfort about Pierre's behavior, energy built. Several mothers, led by Patti—who had two adolescent daughters—wanted to confront Pierre before camp ended. On Friday, as campers were walking to the final work session, Serena and Patti talked. As Serena described that conversation,

> I think I got swept up in the energy and the drama of what was going on. On the way to our last session, Patti told me that both her girls were very uncomfortable around Pierre and felt he had been "spying on them" all week. I said to Patti, really in kind of an off-handed manner, "Well, I agree with them. Pierre just keeps weirding me out with his looks and his side comments to me about how sexy I am."
> Before I knew it, Patti was pushing me to say something. She kept saying, "Serena, someone has got to speak up. The girls are just too uncomfortable to say anything in front of the large group. You need to speak for all of them."
> So that's what happened. Without really thinking about it I got up in front of the group to say that I was really uncomfortable about Pierre and how he treated women all week. Now that I think about it, I feel bad 'cause I never told Pierre that I didn't like what he was doing. I mean, to be honest, for me, his behavior wasn't that big a deal. But after I talked to Patti, I guess I got up 'cause I felt like someone needed to say something. And boy was that the beginning of a whole lot of people saying a whole lot of things nobody had talked about for years!

Generally, the final work session is a time for people to wrap up the week's experience. That year, no one was scheduled to do individual work and campers expected the session to be brief. When the facilitators invited people to share any last comments or concerns about the week, Serena raised her concern about Pierre's behavior. Betty, age 17, followed.

Betty: I'm so glad Serena said something. This has been a really bad week for me. I felt so unsafe and so uncomfortable. Pierre, you do not understand how you come across to people, especially women. Maybe you don't think it is a big deal to look at a woman's body the way you do, but it is for me. [*She cries, and her sister steps forward to speak.*]

Sue: And I don't want anyone thinking, "Oh, that's just Betty and 'cause she was molested when she was little, she thinks every man who looks at her is going to do something sexual." That is not it at all. All of us are uncomfortable with Pierre. He is always standing outside the bathrooms whenever we go to shower. One day, I found him standing in the entrance of the women's bathroom by the pool, and when I said, "Hey, what are you doing?," he made some lame excuse about checking the trash. I mean, what a perv.

[*Other women come forward and speak. Then*]:

Maura: I'm aware of how many people are uncomfortable with what happened this week with Pierre, and I know that many of you have felt unheard during the week. But I'm also concerned that we not start to gang up on one person, even when it's clear he has upset so many people.

Athena [*with startling energy*]: I think the energy you hear and feel isn't just about Pierre. Yeah, I didn't like what he did this week, either, but there is a much larger issue that we are not talking about. I think we need to be honest that Pierre is taking a lot of the upset and betrayal we have all felt for years about Mick and how he has used women in the camp.

[*A momentary shocked silence and a high level of discomfort hangs in the air.*]

Tina: Athena is right. I got up here to talk about Pierre 'cause I agree with Betty, and I don't want her to feel like she is the only one who has those concerns, but Athena has helped me realize that what I am really feeling . . . why we are all so upset about Pierre . . . is 'cause we let all this stuff with Mick go on and on.

[*addressing her mother, who was sitting in front with a stunned expression*], you know it's true, you know what he does. [*Tina cries, and her mother, Yvonne, rushes up to comfort her.*]

Yvonne: Tina is right. We have allowed Mick to operate for years, doing some of the things we are all so outraged with Pierre about. I have never felt comfortable with Mick once Tina told me that he was feeling her up when he hugged her.

[*To her daughter*]: And Tina, I'm so sorry that all I did was tell you to stay out of his way. You were right, we should have done something then.

Audience voices tumbled over each other. Nita came forward and asked people to speak one at a time. She suggested that they address their experiences or reactions to either Pierre or Mick. The chaos lessened, and a growing number of women stood up to take their turn.

Phyllis: Well, I'm another mother who just warned her daughter to avoid Mick. I have had a lot of uncomfortable exchanges with Mick. He has touched me in ways I didn't like and made comments that made me just want to slap him. But it seemed like it was understood at camp that this is the way Mick is, and it was up to us as women to stay out of his way.

Athena: I think a lot of the reason it has gone on is because, let's face it, Mick has been really important to camp. [*Looking directly at Mick*]: And you made it clear, both you and you, Rose, that if we didn't do things your way, then you would just leave camp and we would not have your support anymore.

Athena was the first to speak directly to Rose and Mick, who had remained in their seats throughout the onslaught of words and emotions. Both were shocked and looked almost ill as accusations filled the air. When Athena spoke to them directly, Mick stood and tried to find words to express his shock and outrage.

> Mick: I do not have to put up with this. I will not be accused like this. After all I have done for this group. . . . This never would have happened if Virginia were still alive.
>
> Rose [*standing beside Mick and speaking forcefully*]: Mick, we need to leave. I thought these people were our friends and our family. There is no one here who cares about us and how horrible and hurtful this is to us. Please let's just go. I cannot listen to another word.

Rose had to pull on Mick to get him to leave. It was clear that he would have preferred to stay and defend himself, but she won out and the couple left the session. Their close friends, Marnie and Calvin, got up and told the group that they would go and talk with them. The remaining group became more subdued, and several people began to express remorse about what had just happened.

> Stan: I know the way Mick behaves has upset some people, but I think we should have confronted him differently.
>
> Nelson: That may be true, Stan, but sooner or later, this had to come out. We all know it has been there for years, like a boil about to burst. I think Athena is right. We just couldn't do it until we felt like he had less power over us. And I don't think it's just a coincidence that it happened with Virginia gone and when Eliana had to leave early.
>
> Athena: I'm sorry this all came out as it did and that Mick and Rose feel attacked. But it really is time for camp to deal with this issue. Mick and Rose have had this power too long. We cannot hold Pierre accountable without doing the same thing with Mick.
>
> Anna Marie [Pierre and Pauline's sponsor at camp]: Well, let me tell you I don't know who to be mad at, but *I am furious!* How can we say we are a community who supports every individual and then treat people the way we just treated Pierre and Mick? I mean, never mind that I invited Pierre to camp and he is my cousin, I would feel the same way if I had just met him. He is a person with feelings and

he has just been humiliated in front of his wife and all of you. Do you have any idea how mean and nasty you all have been for the last hour?

Okay, things have happened. So why didn't anyone come to Pierre and just tell him how you feel? What good is all this "trust each other" and "let's be honest about who we are and how we feel" bullshit? How can you say you believe and follow Virginia's principles if not one person could be straight and direct and just say, "Hey, Pierre, knock it off"? Or better yet, maybe check out your assumptions about what he was doing in the first place.

Nita: I think it is important to remember that when someone feels they have been assaulted . . .

Anna Marie: *Assaulted?* Now we're saying Pierre assaulted people? Oh, come on, give me a break. I thought we were talking about Pierre looking at young girls' boobs.

Nita: It would help if you would let me finish. When I say "assaulted," I'm talking about how someone feels—and, yes, even looks can feel like an assault. It is both unfair and unreasonable to expect people who do not feel that they have power, particularly young girls, to confront the person who is offending. I think the community needs to speak for its members, particularly its young and vulnerable members. And when this happens, it's often messy and people's feelings get hurt.

Sean: I think what happened here is a lot more than hurt feelings. I feel this huge renting in the fabric of camp, Mick and Rose are founding members, and we have totally ostracized them with these accusations.

Nelson: Just a minute, Sean, these are not just accusations. There are too many people who share these experiences to minimize them and say they are accusations.

Nita: I agree with Nelson. I think this has gone way beyond accusation. It's important that the community look at how pervasive this behavior has been. Will people who have had exchanges with Mick that have involved inappropriate touching or comments————

Voice from the back: How about inappropriate looks?

Nita: Right, and inappropriate looks. . . . So again, will people who have had exchanges with Mick that involved inappropriate looks, comments, or touching, please raise your hand? [*About a third of the women and many men in the group raised their hands.*]

   This is a lot more than accusations, and something that has needed to be addressed for a long time.

Maura: I agree but I'm really concerned about the way we are addressing it. I'm concerned that here we are at the end of the week and we have opened this huge festering boil, and it needs some emergency attention. I certainly have my feelings about Mick, but I also agree with Anna Marie's concerns. Pierre and his family and Rose and Mick are members of our community, and they deserve our concern and support as well.

Nelson: I agree with Maura. What I suggest is that some of us meet with Mick and Rose. [*Noticing Calvin in the back of the group*]: Calvin, do you know where they are now?

Calvin: Well, they are horribly upset. I left them with Marnie in the kitchen, but I expect they will be packing to leave very soon. They said they will not stay tonight and just want to get away.

Nita: I think it might be good if I talk with them first to see if they want to talk with a smaller group. If they are willing to stay and talk about this with other members of camp, are there people who would be willing to meet with them?

The group agreed with Nita's proposal. Maura, Nelson, and Sean volunteered to meet with Rose and Mick. As they left, Marx stepped to the front of the group and said, "I would like to end this session and then meet with Pierre and Pauline. Will that be okay with you?"

Pierre and Pauline agreed. Given the group's strong emotions and general confusion, Marx brought the session to a dissatisfying close. Members of the larger group wandered off or clustered in smaller groups to continue the discussion.

In a meeting held later in the day, Nita, Marx, and Maura worked to help Pierre and Pauline understand the camp's concern about Pierre's behavior. Throughout the discussion, both Pierre and Pauline insisted they saw no reason why everyone "came so unglued." Their session ended this way:

> Pierre: So I guess the girls didn't like me hanging around them.
>
> Nita: It really is more than hanging around, Pierre. They felt that you were looking at them for sexual gratification.
>
> Pierre: For what?
>
> Maura: That the way you were looking at them turned you on.
>
> Pierre: Oh, well, yeah, I mean some of these girls are really good looking.
>
> Nita: And that is why everyone is so concerned, Pierre. They are girls and you are an adult, and we come here to be together as a family, not to get turned on.
>
> Pauline: Well, you never felt like family to me. I mean, people here are really stuck up. We just never fit in, and now everyone wants to blame Pierre for what that dirty old man did. You people are really a piece of work. I told you, Pierre, any place your cousin likes is bound to be full of weirdos.
>
> Nita: I know this has been a hard week for both of you. I really hope that you will think about what has happened and look at how Pierre's behavior upsets people. You are right, there are problems here that have to do with Mick and what he has done, but it does not mean that Pierre should not listen to what the girls and women have been saying and think about how his actions have affected people here at camp.
>
> Pierre: You know, I've had just about enough of this. I tried to be friendly, that's all. I sure didn't feel anybody up or do the stuff they said Mick did. Still, that little tramp called me a perv. I'm sick of listening to all this bullshit. I just want to get packed and out of here. You're right, Pauline, these people are total weirdos.

Pierre, Pauline, and Anna Marie packed and left camp early the next morning. They have never returned to camp. Mick and Rose refused to meet with anyone. They packed their belongings and left camp that evening.

Nelson described the closing of camp that year:

> It was just surreal. Remember, this all happened on Friday, and Friday night is Skit Night, which is a really big deal for the kids. So

there we are. Mick and Rose are storming off, and the only people they will let near them are Marnie and Calvin. So of course, Marnie and Calvin are upset, and when Marnie and Calvin are upset, then a good half of the camp is upset.

Then Pierre and Pauline stalk off to their tent and just hide away until they leave the next morning. And don't forget about Anna Marie. She is furious, and when Anna Marie gets angry about something—anything—we all know about it. And through it all, the kids are setting up for "Captain Nemo" [an annual skit by the teens]. We went ahead with Skit Night, but let me tell you, it was pretty damned difficult to drum up any enthusiasm.

Maura said:

The next day was Closing, and it just kind of happened. I can't even remember if we had a ceremony. Most of the Committee was still trying to repair the damage from the last session on Friday and the drama that followed. Everyone regretted how the confrontation happened, especially with Mick. Not that it happened, just how it happened . . . and the affect it had on Rose. It was just a horrible, horrible ending.

Although sfc learned a great deal from the "Mick Incident," the damage to the relationship between camp, Mick, and Rose was never repaired. Throughout the following year, the Committee continued its discussion about what happened and wrote letters to Pierre, Pauline, and Anne Marie as well as to Mick and Rose, expressing regret for the manner in which the issue was raised and expressing concern for each of them. Eliana became involved with both the Committee and with Mick and Rose. Although sfc fully acknowledged that the process had been traumatic for all, the community was unwilling to deny or minimize the content of what members had said.

Both Mick and Rose continued to minimize as well as deny most of the accounts made by the women at camp, and no one found a resolution that would allow Mick or Rose to find a way to return to camp.

Community Implications

The move to Camp Loma in 1992 was, in part, a reaction to the Rebellion that occurred after the 1991 camp evacuation and accident. The first year at Camp Loma, the community focused on challenging the status quo of leadership and its decisions, as well as adjusting to the new camp location. The community also began to question whether everyone's needs were being met equally.

The "Mick Incident" represented a significant event in the community's development. The event was triggered by the change in leadership, including the addition of two new therapists, and the change in the camp's location. Without Virginia's authoritarian leadership, the community became more structured and more democratic. Virginia had engendered such trust that no one questioned her decisions about how or how not to address an issue. If she did not see something as a community problem, people thought, maybe it wasn't worth bringing up.

With group leaders who took ownership in the camp's structure, the community began to address problems among its members. Evidence of this lies in the group's initial attempts to address the use of drugs and alcohol at camp as well as confronting the inappropriate behavior of a community founder.

Clearly, the community had been approaching this level of independence for some time. Just as clearly, to achieve total independence, the camp had to address old taboos and sever ties to the old power structure. This could not happen without taking on the power positions of Virginia's Inner Circle. In the climate of silence, which included Virginia's silence, such behavior had characterized many years at Pico Blanco.

Unfortunately, it is not uncommon for those whose needs are being met to exist in a state of ignorance or total oblivion to the unmet needs of others in a group. This may, in part, explain the surprise and outrage expressed by Mick and Rose during the confrontation and their possible inability to integrate the information into their understanding of camp.

Had Virginia been present when this session finally occurred, most long-term campers believe that she would have addressed the issue of victimization in just as supportive a manner. These campers insist that she would not have ignored the same level of outcry and distress from even one member of the community, let alone more than a third of its women.

However, as noted, the community did not seem to feel independent enough or empowered enough to address the boundary issues with a member of the Inner Circle when Virginia was still in a leadership position.

The change factors present during sfc's first year at Camp Loma—i.e. new location, new campers, new leadership structure, and new therapists—represent both the energy of the Foreign Element as well as that of Chaos. Chaos erupted during direct confrontation of the "old guard" and the outcry that ensued. These energies fueled the Rebellion stage of community development that year. The Rebellion stage challenged the Status Quo and identified unmet needs of the community.

Pierre's behavior presented the community with the needed catalyst to identify the unmet needs of many of the camp's females. Year after year, many of the women had experienced a lack privacy, safety, and freedom from harassment. In 1992, camp energy focused on identifying these unmet needs, upsetting the balance of the previously established structure, and changing community expectations.

5

Redefinition and Synergy

Immediately following the 1992 camp and in the months leading up to the 1993 camp, the Committee tried to heal the divisions created within the community by the events at the end of the 1992 camp. For the first time, people began to express their discomfort about both the past as well as what occurred at that camp and began to redefine expectations and parameters of acceptable behaviors.

The chaotic energy of the Rebellion stage at the 1992 camp set the stage for Redefinition, which began immediately after camp, continued through the rest of the year, and lasted into the 1993 camp. The Rebellion stage that occurred during the final year at Pico Blanco and continued through the first year at Camp Loma led the community into the Redefinition Stage.

Because of the chaos in 1992, registration for the 1993 camp was low and added fiscal problems to the litany of concerns facing the camp. The Committee decided to make a concerted effort to recruit new members into the community. Pam Walker, camp president in 1993—along with other campers from Santa Barbara, California— recruited a group of new families from Santa Barbara's home-school community.

In many ways, these families replicated the young families described in Chapter 2. Most came to camp with young children, and as a group, they shared a common philosophy about education and child rearing. But they also differed from existing campers. Most were new to the Satir philosophy and therapeutic methods. Their openness and enthusiasm helped balance the rather bruised parts of the community that survived the two years of Chaos that preceded the 1993 camp.

It took several more years to resolve the Chaos stage. Some resolution came about simply because the people most involved in the conflict left camp. The new families in 1993 had no experience with the past traumas, which further dissipated the chaotic energy. The lead therapist also returned to camp in 1993 and brought a sense of stability to the therapeutic team.

Boundary Issues and Sex at Camp

At the same time, the chaos born in 1992 affected camp significantly. Two fundamental issues had surfaced: the community's holding of a "family secret" (regarding Mick's sexual behavior) and the ability of individuals as well as the community as a whole to set and maintain boundaries that provide safety as well as comfort for all involved. As part of its attempt to address these issues, the Committee and the therapists agreed to look at how the community viewed and wanted to deal with boundary issues, especially around sex. At its quarterly meetings held between the 1992 and 1993 camps, the Committee discussed the confusion about boundaries as one of the many reasons that the community had kept Mick's behavior secret for so many years.

The Committee and the therapeutic team decided to work with the camp community to assure that boundaries would be clear at camp. All three facilitators attended the Committee's November 1993 meeting to review events at the 1992 camp as well as how the crisis had developed over the years. The Committee and the therapists planned interventions to help address the issue now that the camp secret had been revealed.

For the 1993 camp, the Committee decided to use a theme: the way men and women perceive as well as misperceive sexual communication, particularly sexual comments and nonverbal sexual language. The focus was on how men and women relate around sexual issues while living together at camp. With the help of the therapists, the Committee decided to foster an open dialogue about sex and relationships between men and women and to have the community define as well as redefine boundaries in the sFc community.

The following discussion is fictional, albeit based on events at that camp.

> Eliana: One of the things that I learned during the year when I
> met with Mick and Rose and then the Committee is that

we need to work on how we communicate with one another as sexual beings. We all have learned that there have been sexual exchanges that have made people uncomfortable for many years. We now know that many people did not want or appreciate these sexual exchanges, yet they were not able to discuss their feelings openly.

Virginia taught us that life is messy. She taught us that we will make mistakes as we live our life journey because we are human and we are always learning. But Virginia also said that after we make our mistakes, we need to take out our broom and clean up the mess we made. And that is what we hope to do today. We want to take the time to learn from our mistakes and to start cleaning things up so that we can all feel safe and be more open and clear in our communication. We want to be able to learn about our own boundaries, and then we want to learn how to let others know about our boundaries as individuals and as a community.

Nita: I want to talk about how physical intimacy can be a challenge for people, particularly here at camp. We come together in this often highly charged atmosphere to share our most intense longings and deepest experiences. This sharing then leads to intense feelings of intimacy.

The intensity of these feelings, particularly if they are followed by expressions of physical intimacy, can cause confusion and sometimes conflict. Some people are more comfortable with the physical expression of intimacy and are open to being touched. Others have much stronger boundaries in this area and are uncomfortable with physical contact. Some people become uncomfortable when another person enters his or her personal space.

We all bring our own history and experience with physical intimacy to camp. We have our own way of defining what is and is not acceptable physical intimacy. For some people, a hug may mean the initiation of sexual intimacy. For others, it may simply be an expression of emotional intimacy with no sexual meaning. And there are people who cannot tolerate any type of physical touch. This may be because of his or her early history, when any physical contact led to unwanted sexual activity. It is important that we remember that each of us responds to intimacy and physical contact in a unique manner and in a way that may differ from another person.

After the therapists introduced the subject, campers discussed their feelings about intimacy and physical contact. Differences between men and women as well as between generations quickly become apparent. The group discussed appropriate and inappropriate responses to physical appearance, clothes, and sexual behaviors. Members also talked about how sexual messages between men and women can be misinterpreted. After discussing general issues such as comments about a person's body or appearance, the young women in the group become more direct.

> Lizabeth: I think the thing that bugs me the most is how men are always looking at women's breasts. I feel that I should be able to wear a tee shirt and not have to worry about whether it's going to make some guy feel horny.
>
> Robin: I guess I understand what you mean but, come on, when women—and I mean girls as well as women—start wearing tight tee shirts without a bra and their nipples show, well, what do you expect?
>
> Athena [*in a clear and somewhat frustrated tone*]: What we expect is to be able to wear what we want, what feels comfortable, and not be treated like some sex object. I don't wear tee shirts without a bra to get attention; I wear them because they are comfortable. If that turns on some man, well, that's his problem, not mine.

The energy in the group grew and tension filled the air as several of the men, particularly those of the older generation, stuck with the argument that men are just responding to what they see. They expressed the opinion that if women do not want that type of attention, then they should not wear revealing clothes.

> Alisa: I think this discussion is more a difference between generations than a difference between men and women. I was taught, and I am sorry to say I also accepted, that if I wore some type of tight sweater or skirt and got unwanted comments or glances from men, I was responsible for causing them. I find it wonderful that the young women of our community are so clear about their right to be who

they are and wear the clothes they want. I totally agree that it is not their problem if men respond to their outfits by getting turned on. I think it just shows how far we have come in allowing women to be women rather than sex objects.

Fred: I agree with Alisa, but I also think women need to understand that a lot of men need time to learn new behaviors, and we don't always do that so well. I remember when I was complimenting a young woman and said something like, "You look very attractive. I bet all the boys will notice you when you walk in the room."

She responded to what I thought was a great compliment by telling me, "You know, you could have stopped after you said I look attractive." I thought about that for a long time and realized that it was true. I didn't need to add the part about the boys, but it was just the way we complimented girls when I was growing up. Now that it has been pointed out to me, I am more aware of how often there is an undertone of male-oriented sexuality in things I was saying.

Athena: I know we probably need to be more patient, but a lot of times I just don't feel it's my job to make men aware of their chauvinism or their harassment. I remember when I was being harassed by this guy on my first job. I was told that I had to tell him to stop first, or I couldn't file a complaint. I was so pissed I just quit. Why should I have to tell someone to stop trying to feel me up on the elevator?

Susana: That is such bullshit. Then men wonder why we get so defensive about this sexual stuff. You know, when I come to camp, I never think about having men come on to me. I come to camp to be with family. I love having all the guys that I grew up with here as friends and that I can just be me when I hang out with them. As for the older men, well, after last summer, I can tell you, anyone who comes here and tries to be sexual with any of us is going to be in for big trouble.

As the young women began to dominate it, most of the men retreated from the discussion. Many of the older women talked about their experiences growing up in a different culture, but the discussion between men and women ended. Later in the day, however, the men's group continued the discussion. In that setting, the men were able to discuss how difficult it was for them to approach women. Most of the men, particularly those over forty, acknowledged they were still learning how to relate in ways that women—particularly the younger women—would not misinterpret. Later, a 60-year-old male camper said:

> I certainly didn't feel like we solved the problem that year. In many ways, the men just shut up and listened. Nevertheless, the discussions did make us more aware of how our lack of awareness can impact women, and I guess that made things get better.

A female camper remarked:

> I was surprised how willing the community was to talk about sexual issues and how men and women relate. After all, this was just one year after the big confrontation with Mick and Pierre, which followed years of people not saying anything about pretty blatant behavior by at least one member of the community.

Another woman said that in 1993, her first year at SFC:

> . . . it was clear there was a lot of energy about sexual issues in camp. At first, I was taken aback by all this concern about sex, but once I heard about what had been happening in past camps, it made more sense. One of the things that made me feel so good about camp was the way the community took what seemed like a horrible event and made it into a learning experience for everyone, even those of us who were new that year.

Her husband spoke in a similar vein:

> Our introduction to camp was pretty challenging because we started the year after the Big Incident. I must admit I spent a lot of time wondering, "What the heck am I doing here?" There was an undercurrent about things I knew nothing about. By the end of the week, I felt more comfortable, and I sure learned a lot about how men and women relate!

Although this discussion in 1993 did not solve all issues between men and women, it did help open the dialogue. It also demonstrated to community members that sexual issues are party of the larger issue of setting boundaries and feeling safe in the community. Through this dialogue, campers were not only given permission but were encouraged to set boundaries for themselves and to speak up when they felt that someone was not respecting those boundaries.

Sexual Diversity

Issues tied to sexuality exist in every intentional community and create challenges related to boundaries and also to sexual diversity. Families headed by lesbian parents have been a part of sfc for many years. Interestingly, when the camp's first lesbian couple decided to have a child together in the mid 1980s, Virginia advised against their decision, counseling that their child would resent them. One of the moms said later:

> I was taken back by Virginia's resistance to our decision to have a child, but in some ways she just reflected the professional attitudes toward gay parenting at that time. I know had she lived she would have changed her attitude, just as most mental health professionals have changed.

The community's response to male homosexual members and to open sexuality has been more guarded. One long-time male camper said:

> Over the years, sfc has become more traditional and less open in its sexual attitudes and practices. When I shared with the men's group and then the community at large that I am bisexual, I felt a distancing in my relationships with the men. I think, like society at large, this community is less threatened by women's sexuality and much more uncomfortable with male homosexuality.

Anaka, a female camper, recounted:

> My husband and I have an open marriage, and I know that makes some people in camp uncomfortable. I like this community, but it is not a place where I feel who I am sexually is accepted.

As society as a whole has changed attitudes about sex and sexual practices since the early 1970s, so has sfc. As a result, during this period of Redefinition, the community has reexamined how it deals with sexual practices in camp. The following story illustrates how the sfc community responded to Anaka and her husband, Johan, who had been open about their sexual practices. Anaka asked to address the community. Carl, then camp president, addressed the fifteen members of the Pulse Committee.

Carl: Anaka is here to make a request. Go ahead, Anaka.

Anaka: Thanks, Carl. I feel a little awkward about this, so I hope you will bear with me while I try to explain what I'm asking for. Actually, I'm here representing myself as well as Johan and Cole [*another camper*]. So . . . we're requesting time at a session to talk about our relationship.

Serena: Whose relationship?

Anaka: Well, I think you know that Johan and I have an open marriage, and during this year Cole and I have become lovers and————

Sondra: Well, I don't really see what that has to do with any of us!

Carl: Why don't we let her finish her request before we draw any conclusions? Go on, Anaka.

Anaka: Well, in a way, you are right, Sondra, it really is mostly our business. But this is the first time that Johan and I have been involved with someone who is another camper, and we just want to be open and comfortable about that relationship. We would prefer to talk about it with people so they understand what this relationship means to us and to our families.

Anaka and Johan have two daughters, and Cole has one adult daughter, all of whom are also at camp.

Sondra: I don't see why you have to bring it up at all. I mean, we all know you have an open relationship, and I think you know not everyone is comfortable with that, but that is up to you. Why make an issue of it here at camp?

Anaka [*becoming frustrated*]: Because we want to be able to help people understand who we are and what all of this means to us. We know there are people who have questions about what it means to be in an open relationship, and we want to be able to talk about that and answer their questions. What we do not want is to feel judged or gossiped about. We all know that there have been other relationships in camp that were not talked about openly, but everybody did talk about it behind their backs. We just don't want that to happen to us.

Glen [*a therapist*]: I appreciate your being so open and willing to discuss this with the Pulse Committee, Anaka. At the same time, I know that we need as much session time as we can get for the people who have already asked to work. You aren't asking to do work about this, are you?

Anaka [*laughing nervously*]: No, we are fine with our relationship. We just want to be open with people at camp.

Eliana: Well, how about we do this. You can announce at a session meeting that you want to share with people your new relationship and then anyone who is interested in hearing about it can join you, say, tonight after dinner? [*Turning to the group*]: How does that sound? [*Most group members nod in agreement and seem almost relieved about this proposal.*]

Anaka [*less pleased*]: Well, if that's the only way we can do it, I guess that's how it will be. So, we can make the announcement at session this morning?

Carl: Okay, Glen, you'll make sure that they have time to do that?

As that morning's work session began, Glen announced to the group that before beginning the scheduled work, Anaka wanted to make an announcement. Anaka, Johan, and Cole all came forward.

Anaka: Actually, this is an announcement from the three of us. We want to invite anyone who is interested to join us after dinner tonight here at the session area to talk about our relationship.

Johan: The three of us have joined together as a family, and we would like to share what that means to us and to answer any questions you might have.

Cole: I just want to add that I'm very proud of how we have joined together and hope that you will come and learn more.

The threesome sits down. No one responds, and Glen moves on to begin the session. Anaka said later:

> It was so awkward. I mean, we make this announcement but we can't really say much because we agreed to do that only with people who "wanted to hear about it." I just think the Pulse Committee was

incredibly uptight and uncomfortable about the topic and us. I was surprised that so many people did in fact come to hear us.

Cole said:

> I know Anaka wanted to have the discussion during a session, but I was relieved that we did it on our own with people who chose to come and meet with us. To tell the truth, I didn't trust the therapists to handle things the way I knew we could. I wanted us to be in complete control, to tell the story our way. In the end, a lot of people came to hear it . . . which was really nice.

Following dinner, a group of about forty campers, almost all adults, came to the session area. Cole, Anaka, and Johan had decided to each take turns telling their story and then to answer questions.

> Anaka: I'm really glad so many people decided to come. I'm a little nervous. Where to begin? Well, I guess what I want to say is that about six months ago, I asked Cole if he would be interested in having a sexual relationship with me. Johan and I had begun to explore an open marriage, and I realized that I wanted to get more involved with someone on an emotional as well as sexual level, and to do that, I wanted to be involved with someone I knew and who knew my family. Johan was supportive, so I called Cole and he and I agreed to meet and talk about it more.

> Cole: I must admit I was pretty surprised when she called. I knew that they had been exploring an open marriage, and I had shared my experiences with Johan in men's group, but it never occurred to me that Anaka would want to get involved with me. So we talked on the phone, and I guess at first it just seemed complicated. I mean, we live three states apart and we really only see each other at camp. At that point, I was exploring my own sexuality and exploring my interest in men as well as women, and I wasn't really sure that was what Anaka would want.

> Anaka: So at first, it didn't seem like it would work but then Cole came to our area and he called, and it was at this really difficult time for us.

> Johan: See, I had broken both my arm and leg a month earlier, and we were really struggling with all kinds of problems

and of course emotions. I was angry at being so limited physically and having to depend on Anaka so much. And my business wasn't doing well, and I just felt awful. I guess you would think that isn't a great time for your wife to invite another man into the house, but it just worked for us. Cole just brought such a healing energy into our home. He helped with the kids and was so wonderful with both Anaka and me.

Anaka: And we found that we could share our sexuality as a threesome as well as a couple, and that was just a total surprise.

Cole: Definitely a surprise for all of us. I don't think any of us planned it that way, but that is what happened. And now I try to visit with the family at least every couple of months, and I feel part of their lives and they are a part of mine.

[*Gradually, people who had been listening involved themselves in the discussion.*]

Phyllis: What I'm wondering about are the kids. Do they know what is going on?

Anaka: Well, you know our girls are young, so we certainly don't involve them in a discussion of our sex lives. But they do know that Cole has become a part of our family and that both Johan and I love him and want him to visit and be with us. I think they have some awareness of this relationship being special.

Beth, my oldest, said the other day when we were talking about Cole coming to visit: "You know, Mom, you and Dad always do things just a little different than most parents, and I like that. I think I'm lucky to have another parent who loves me." I just felt so proud that she sees how including someone else in the family adds to the love available to all of us.

Cole: I certainly have talked to Janet [his daughter] about it. She knows that I'm bisexual and, although I think it is hard for her, sometimes I know that we can talk about it, and she knows that I will always be honest with her. She enjoys the younger kids and seems even happier to have a sibling relationship with them.

Johan: For me, the kids are an important part of what I get from this relationship. Like Beth said, there is just a lot more love in the house. We are able to satisfy each other more and therefore to make ourselves more available to the kids. With our kids, we aren't as open about the sex as Cole has been with Janet, but we will be when they become older.

Stefan: Are you concerned about what others—like us here at camp—think about what you are doing?

Anaka: Sure, there is a part of me that is worried about being judged. I guess it might have been easier to keep this private. What's most important, though, is being honest about the relationship and not having people wonder what's going on. We don't want to be sneaking around, and we don't want people gossiping about us. If people choose to judge us, well, I guess that's up to them. I won't necessarily like it, but at least I know they have the real story about what we are doing and why.

Cole: This community means a great deal to me. Therefore, it is very important that I am able to be very honest about who I am and about whom I love. I'm not looking for everyone to approve or agree with me. I just want people to respect me and my choices, even if the choices aren't ones they would make.

Johan: I really don't worry much about what other people think. But my kids are here, and I want this community to respect our family and not have us become fodder for the gossip machine. I feel when people understand who we are and know that we are not only careful but loving in the relationships we have, I think the rest will just fall into place.

Paul: I must admit I wasn't sure how I felt when Anaka came this morning and asked to talk to the community about this. I feel much clearer and have a great deal of respect for your willingness to share this part of your life with us. I'm concerned about how our community reacts to people who practice or believe things that are not part of the mainstream. Your being willing to share your story helps us all grow in our understanding of different ways that people choose to love. I think you have done a wonderful job of explaining your relationship and your feelings for each other, and I want to say thank you.

New as well as old campers made similar remarks, and the meeting ended on a very positive and surprisingly low-key note. Johan said later:

> I was overwhelmed by the response we got. There were people that I thought would never come to even hear what we had to say, and they not only came and listened but then they stood up and made such caring, supportive comments. It made me so glad that we came forward to discuss things.

Cole concurred:

> It went better than I could hope. Moreover, it was interesting because ever since then, our involvement with each other has just been a non-issue at camp. I don't have any sense of being judged or looked down on or rejected. I still feel that camp has very traditional values about sex and great ambivalence about gay men, in particular, but I feel totally accepted there in this relationship.

Unwanted Sexual Advances

Although the sfc community supports sexual diversity, it continues to struggle with sexual issues. Not surprisingly, the intensity of the emotional intimacy fostered in the community sometimes leads to sexual intimacy among campers. These connections have led to both new and changing relationships among campers. They also have resulted in challenges to the community, most particularly how to respond to people who make unwanted sexual advances.

Campers are aware that all of the therapists and the Executive Committee are available to respond to any level of concern that anyone may be feeling about sexual issues. Because the issue of unwanted sexual advances brings back memories of past chaos, such reports receive speedy and confidential handling. sfc does not have explicit rules or policies regarding sexual conduct, and some campers experience inappropriate conduct during camp. The community has become more proactive when a camper raises the problem, and the Committee as well as the therapists continue to encourage community discussions about the importance of setting, maintaining, and respecting boundaries.

Not all campers find this approach helpful, however. Not everyone who has been offended or has endured unwanted advances makes a complaint, and the community cannot be certain that it is always aware of all violations. Although the community confronts people who cross boundaries and makes them aware that such behavior has been seen and needs to stop, there is no way to monitor future behavior. As the community continues to discuss the issue, it hopes individuals will be more willing to come forward and get support to address the problem, rather than choosing to leave camp to avoid the issue.

The Drug and Alcohol Crisis

In addition to boundary issues, this period of Redefinition also dealt with the use of alcohol and drugs at camp. In 1996, members of the Committee raised the issue at their November 9 meeting. The minutes report:

> Three members of the Board [Committee] reported direct knowledge of the use of marijuana during camp. We reviewed our published policies, which prohibit the use of such substances. We urged those who observe marijuana use to deal directly with the offender, and reaffirmed that we will formally support those who observe marijuana use and intervene.

As happens with complex issues, the members of the Committee took one position in November and revisited the same issue at both the March and May 1997 meetings. By March, it had become clear that the drug issue was a symptom of other issues within the Committee and the community as a whole. At that meeting, the Committee addressed the underlying issues. Edited slightly for clarity, the March 1997 minutes said:

> Committee needs to be more open about feelings of its members;
> Unresolved issues are very upsetting and have resulted in
>   people leaving camp with unresolved feelings.
> How do we take care of people at camp?
> There is a betrayal of trust among Committee members.
> We are slow to process internal camp issues. We need to take a
>   risk and discuss issues such as drug use in camp.
> There is a lack of safety in camp in discussing feelings.
> How do we keep anxiety level down at camp?
> Camp has gone from being matriarchal to trusting group wisdom.

With the assistance of a group facilitator, the Committee opened a dialogue that allowed all Committee members to be both honest and constructive about feelings among members. For one intense meeting, chaotic energy reigned as the president resigned and the Committee had to deal with the confusion and upset created by strong feelings. A current Committee member recounted:

> I wasn't on the Committee that year but came by to see people during lunch to pick up a cheesecake I had won at the auction at the last camp. Well, I knew it must have been one difficult meeting, because they had eaten my cheesecake, and it wasn't even lunchtime! Several people told me they wondered if camp would survive this year. I tell you, it took me a lot more years before I would even consider joining the Committee after I saw how people were struggling that year.

Despite the almost desperate feelings just described, the Committee worked through its issues. The vice president stepped into the president's role. The Committee worked with the facilitator throughout the afternoon, went to dinner as a group, and finally addressed its business issues late in the evening. Despite low registration, resignation of the Committee secretary and the camp cook, as well as many conflicted relationships, the Committee met again by May and put plans for the 1997 camp into full swing. They hired a new cook and asked the camp secretary to rescind his resignation.

Relationship discussions continued. Committee meeting minutes of May 1997 report:

> We delved into the serious breaches in personal relationships which now exist among several members of the community, and we examined how those breaches occurred, and what is preventing their healing. We traced the pattern of how interpersonal problems have been managed in our community, going back several years. We achieved broad agreement that the way we have handled these occasions is inconsistent with our expressed values.

At the same meeting, the Committee again addressed how it wanted to deal with violations of its stated policy on marijuana use at camp. The minutes explain:

> The issue of illicit substance usage was revisited. During the discussion, we acknowledged how terribly damaging the use of

marijuana has been to our community. We, as the leadership, are not of one mind on this issue. How we are to respond to this remains problematic. In the discussion, a continuum of priorities became evident, ranging from the individualistic, placing priority on individual prerogatives on the one hand, but some others placed priority on a concern for the entire community.

We have lots of fears and anxieties, but scant information. It was generally agreed that if an individual discovers the use of illegal substances, or the misuse or abuse of legal substances, it will be dealt with at the person-to-person level. If that intervention succeeds, nothing further needs to be done. But if the intervention does not result in the desired change, then members of the leadership shall be informed, and the response will be based on a case by case assessment of the appropriate action. This was a grave discussion, a struggle which was not easy for any of the participants.

In the same way that the community is not always successful addressing boundary violations, it continues to struggle over how to deal with violations of the alcohol and drugs policy. The community as a whole has discussed the use of alcohol, particularly by the teens, as well as use of drugs by any camper. It was not until 2002, however, that the Committee distributed a written policy regarding the camp's position on alcohol and drugs. The policy clarified that SFC does not allow the use of illegal substances or underage drinking. The Committee mailed this policy to all campers age 10 years and older, asking people not to attend camp if they could not follow the policy.

At the same time, the community remains divided about whether to use punitive actions with repeat offenders. SFC focuses on prevention, early identification, treatment, and support for members who have a drug or alcohol problem. The camp continues to respond to these issues by addressing each situation on an individual basis. Debate continues regarding the best way to support individuals while protecting the community as a whole.

Development of a Mission Statement

The ten annual camps held between 1993 and early 2003 span the community's middle years and its development through the stages of Redefinition and Synergy, ending with movement toward Ennui. A critical transition came in 1996–97, moving from the chaos of the confronting Pierre and Mick to the chaos within the Committee when individual Committee members confronted each other. As a result of these confrontations, the community returned to the Definition stage at the 1997 camp. In that process, the community as a whole participated in a work session to write a community mission statement. Although sfc had operated until then with an informal statement of purpose developed by the Committee, this was the first formal mission statement written and approved by the entire community. Posted at each camp and given to all new members in the sfc Handbook, this statement reads:

> Satir Family Camp is a community in which every individual from infant to elder is known appreciated and respected for his or her unique contributions and inherent goodness.
> Camp is an evolving multicultural community, where each person and families of all kinds are supported and encourage to deepen their communication and connections with one another. With the support of fellow campers, and the assistance of professional guidance in the Satir tradition, the opportunity for personal and family growth is always available.
> Everyone collaborates in the running of camp to provide a safe and healthy environment for sharing, learning, playing, stillness and solitude.
> We seek to explore and expand our individual and group humanity and environmental consciousness at camp and within our larger world family.

This mission statement reflects the community's current as well as future growth. New definitions stressed the importance of a multicultural community as well as a focus on environmental consciousness. The mission statement also restated the community's commitment to Satir principles, philosophies, and methods by providing a place for personal and family growth.

Even with the success of the 1997 camp and the re-establishment of community stability, the Committee continued to work with a facilitator throughout 1998 to achieve a new status quo within the Committee. At the June 1997 Committee meeting, held during the annual camp, the Committee set an agenda for a special two-day meeting in November that would include a full-day facilitated meeting regarding "work on individual and group issues that have hampered our ability to effectively communicate and to conduct regular sfc business" (sfc Committee minutes, June 1997). Such an agenda is indicative of a community with newfound energy to make changes to help itself grow in new and interesting ways.

SFC moved into Synergy at this point, leaving behind the stage of Redefinition. A new focus existed within the Committee, and as a result within the community, on ways to make use of new structure, new expectations, and new resources. This focus stimulated growth and development. The Committee took on challenges that it had previously left with little or no formal evaluation. As is consistent with the stage of Synergy, the Committee began functioning truly as an extension of the community. It worked on developmental issues that no longer centered on basic needs and logistics but on the more subtle and complex issues of relationships and emotional resources within the community.

Leadership Issues: "Big Ducks" and "Little Ducks"

Camp leadership from the late 1980s through the 1990s also affected how the community developed and grew. During the change from Pico Blanco to Camp Loma, several dominant and effective women led SFC. Their leadership was critical to the organization's ability to survive the trauma of the evacuation and accident as well as the confrontation and fallout from the first year at Camp Loma. One member of the Committee commented:

> After Virginia left, camp was dominated and directed by several strong women. They provided excellent leadership, but their style was to go ahead and make decisions and then come to the Committee to get support for that decision from the group. It was different from Virginia's leadership because they listened to others' opinions and often changed their viewpoints when others provided input but still they were the dominant force in camp.

During this period, the camp had one president for over five years. Despite the Committee's request that she remain president as long as she wanted, she recognized the need for a change in leadership and resigned after serving five years. Following that, the Committee set a two-year term for each future president.

Subsequent presidents have had differing styles of leadership. In general, they were less dominant than the first president, causing the Committee as well as the community to reshape its relationships with the camp leaders. In many ways, the Committee grew in strength, particularly when some of the presidents struggled in that role. As one Committee member said:

> Things certainly go smoother when the president is a strong leader and well organized.. Since we tend to process things to death, we need a strong leader who can keep us focused and help us reach consensus. It is also essential that the president follow up after meetings to make sure the decisions get carried out. But even when the president has not been strong or effective, the Committee has benefited because members of the Committee have stepped in and become more involved. No question that when more people are active, the Committee becomes stronger. I think we learned to work better as a Committee when we are not able to depend on just one or two people to do all the work. I believe we have become a stronger as a community was well.

As effective as the leadership was during the years of Rebellion and its inherent chaos, the Committee also contributed to the community's feelings of inclusion and exclusion. That added to members' dissatisfaction and drove the community's entrance into Redefinition. The period of the mid-1980s to mid-1990s has often been called the time of the "Big Ducks" and "Little Ducks," terms that symbolize the strong undercurrents felt throughout the community. As one camper explained:

> You always knew if you were a "Big Duck" or a "Little Duck." The Big Ducks were always listened to and had all the information. The Little Ducks usually did not know what was going on to begin with, and when they did try to express an opinion, it was generally ignored. Much of what happened at camp during those early years at Camp Loma happened because of who you were or who you were friends with rather than because of what the group wanted or thought should happen. I guess that kind of leadership started with Virginia and just continued with the leaders that came after her. And in many ways, that was okay with most people. The Big Ducks cared about camp and made sure things happened, while most of the Little Ducks enjoyed just following along and having their one week at camp.

A Committee member said:

> The part I found hard was the unspoken stuff that went on during those years. There was a lot of gossiping and kind of two-faced stuff happening. In many ways, it was a carry-over from Virginia. She was the consummate professional when she worked with people; but

when she was just Virginia, she could really dish the gossip, and she sure did that at camp. For many years after Virginia left, that style still operated. The community would meet as a group and good things would be said and done, and then we would all get together during meals or in our tents or at night and we would all gossip about each other. It was a hard habit to break.

Another member of the Committee said:

Now that the Committee is less dominated by a few strong personalities, other people have been more willing to confront issues. I think the Big Duck/Little Duck issue is much less important now. Not that it has gone away, it just feels different.

A long-term camper reflected:

Camp is really all about inclusion and exclusion. Not too surprising, in an organization that was created because people want to be part of a community. The issue was much stronger when Virginia was at camp because she had favorites and they got treated differently from the rest of the group. They were the original Big Ducks. Then, after Virginia left, we had a period when a few people dominated most decision making at camp and the Big Ducks/ Little Ducks thing became a focus for community process.

But this time it was different. The so-called Big Ducks were really concerned about the issue, and we addressed it together. The Committee did a work session at camp about how they related to each other, and that helped all of us talk about how people relate and what it means to have power or to feel powerless in this community. The issue never goes away. It is, after all, a family-of-origin issue. So if your issue is feeling rejected or excluded, then you are always on the lookout for exclusion, and you are going to feel it even in a community like ours, where inclusion is a key part of our mission.

And there is also the issue that it is very hard to confront people in a community where you want everyone to feel included and to be happy. Being willing to confront the negative behaviors in other members takes a lot of strength.

Another veteran camper observed:

It's been hard being in a group where people are reluctant to confront each other. For many years, people at sfc have had problems being honest and direct with each other. We so want to support and care for each other that we struggle with the really hard part of telling someone that we don't like what they are doing or that we don't think what they are doing is right or helpful. And that is what I tried to do, and I think I got identified as the person who was the shit disturber. But speaking my truth is what camp is all about for me. I don't come to camp for a summer vacation. I come to camp to be real about me and about the people I love and care for in this community. So I confront what is happening and what is going on and say what I see.

For many years, I felt a deep connection, and it kept drawing me back to camp. I don't feel it as much now, and I'm not really sure why, except fewer people are willing to be as real and as deep in their relationships as we once were at camp.

Building Community: Jobs at Camp

The way SFC has approached jobs at camp also reflects how the community has grown and changed over the years. From its inception, SFC has depended on campers for most of the work needed to support the organization and the weeklong encampment. Volunteer labor has been the key to keeping the costs of camp within an affordable range, particularly for young families. During camp, all community members age 7 to 70 perform jobs, from wiping tables (for those under age 10) to preparing meals and washing up, cleaning latrines, recycling, supervising activities at the pool, and supervising the daily Children's Program. One camper recalled:

> The first year I went camp, I didn't understand the sign-up sheet and managed to sign my family up to do dinner dishes every night of the week. Finally, our sponsor's family took pity on us and helped out so we could get to Skit Night on Friday. Let me tell you, I always check what and how I sign up for, after that experience.

Despite new camper compliance, not everyone gets into the spirit of doing the work. Without some type of monitoring, jobs were not done and certain people did not pull their weight. After several camps at which the problem approached a crisis level, the Committee created the job of "Camp Nag." Each year, one camper— usually a Committee member—has the enviable position of finding campers who forget or choose not to do their jobs, and getting them to work.

Sometimes the Nag was a person with a sense of humor and gentle persuasion, but on several occasions, the assigned Nag embodied the name. Getting jobs done then became more contentious and less friendly.

About that time, a new camper volunteered to be the Nag and brought a new approach to the role as well as to the way that jobs could be incorporated into community development:

> I view the jobs at camp as opportunities for people to participate in building our community, rather than just a way to get the work done. As a result, I viewed the purpose of the Nag differently than most people. As Nag, I saw my role as enabling each person to complete the tasks they signed up for. One way I did this was to give out reminders about the jobs people had signed up for on that day. I used cards and had the kids distribute them to the adults who had jobs that day. This helped get the kids involved and even created a little dialogue between the kids and the adults. When someone did forget, I just let the process happen, and people stepped up and helped and the work got done with a lot less negative energy.

Rather than avoiding them, campers now do jobs as a matter of community pride. Since shifting the way it uses the Nag, sfc has better integrated the jobs into the fabric of the community. During subsequent camps, people have signed up early and often, and jobs have been completed, if not by the person who signed up, then by others who have become aware that a job is uncovered. Campers now see jobs as part of their commitment to camp and its success. It is not a perfect system, but the slight shift in approach and philosophy has gone a long way to making the whole issue a sign of community growth rather than a struggle for survival.

Creating the Camp Nag is a good example of the work done in the stage of Synergy. In earlier stages, it was unusual to have to remind community members to complete jobs. Without completing those jobs—e.g., food, shelter, and safety—the community could not survive. In the new setting of Camp Loma, however, these basic necessities were not critical, and the community focused less energy on survival. The evolution of the Camp Nag role and the Committee tasks that developed over the middle years indicate how the community began to examine resources, relationship, and communication of expectations in a new way.

For many years members of the Committee also did the work required to both open and close camp. These two tasks involve intense effort and a lot of hard work that is often done more effectively by a small work force. In addition, the time spent working as a small group allowed Committee members to strengthen their ties and commitments to each other. For years, they were almost reluctant to share this time with others. However, the tasks required to open and close camp changed as the community became more complex. New tasks—such as setting up and dismantling specialized equipment as well as the camp recycling and compost program—increased the Committee's burden.

During the Committee's discussion of how to use jobs to enhance community building, members decided to add camp closure to the list of jobs for all campers. Now, rather than twenty people working to restore the campgrounds to pre-sfc condition, the entire community pitches in and participates in the last job at camp. Committee members have yet to relinquish the time they spend together setting up camp, but they are more aware of how the camp as a whole benefits from increased responsibility for the running of camp.

The Therapeutic Program

The therapeutic program has also grown and changed since Virginia left and through the late 1990s. Early in this period, the Committee examined how camp uses the therapists as well as how the Committee and therapists work together. The Committee was concerned that some issues were not being addressed effectively because it was not always clear whether it was better for the therapists or the Committee to respond. Discussing these concerns led to further questions about the role and responsibilities of therapists at camp. According to the sfc Committee minutes of November 1997, these questions included:

- To what extent should the facilitators be regarded as part of the community?
- Should we [the Committee] maintain more frequent contact with them; if so, how?
- Should we continue the policy of sending them the minutes of our meetings?
- How much control should the Committee and/or facilitators [therapists] exercise over camp?

Laura Dodson, the lead therapist, became ill during this time and recruited Russ and Karen Haber, a married couple, to work with Tom and Maureen Graves during her absence. When Laura returned, the Committee decided to have all five therapists remain on the team. The Committee also appointed a member of the Executive Committee to serve as liaison between the Committee and the therapeutic team. Having a liaison to communicate with the therapists and address their concerns has helped the Committee, the camp, and the therapists resolve issues as they arise. It also has enhanced the relationships among all three groups. As one sfc therapist sees it,

> When I came to sfc, I had a different focus than the therapists who had come before me. I'm trained in Satir methods and I enjoy the therapeutic work, but my real interest is in developing the community. For me, the therapeutic client is the community at large. Yes, we [the therapists] provide therapeutic services to all parts of that community. But when we do our planning and our assessment, we are responsible to the community as a whole and in particular to the Committee, which is the body that hires us.
>
> I think the therapists who were part of camp after Virginia left began with a different focus. At that time, the therapists continued making many of the governance decisions as well as the therapeutic decisions .It has been challenging for both the therapists and the community to let go of that original relationship. Because I came to sfc after the transition from Pico Blanco, I have been able to work from a different perspective.
>
> The things I most enjoy about camp are the ways we build an intentional community through our daily activities. The basketball games, the ping pong games, working together, eating together are all parts of how we grow as a community. The informal parts of camp life are as important to the community growth as the formal work that we do at Temperature Reading or at sessions.

Providing therapeutic services at sfc is not an easy or lucrative assignment. The therapists work almost 24 hours a day in an environment that offers little time or space for privacy or respite. Five days of the week, therapists provide services to specialized groups (children, teens, young adults, women, men, and special-interest) as well as facilitating at least one general work session. In addition, the therapists attend a daily planning meeting with the camp's leaders to discuss issues arising in camp. Therapists also make themselves available to support individuals and groups outside of the formal therapy groups and Committee meetings; and to consult with camp leaders regarding community issues on an as-needed basis. The community expects therapists to camp at the campgrounds and to participate in community activities.

As the Committee and the therapists' roles became clearer, the team of therapists has separated slightly from the community. They camp together and have built in time to meet as a team, discuss their approach to issues, and support each other during the intensity of the week-long therapeutic marathon.

The Collapsing Camper

Just as they have recognized the need to increase their own support, the therapists have also had to deal with how to support individuals while fostering and protecting the community's growth. A significant issue in a therapeutic community is how to deal with individuals or families who appear to have greater needs than the community can support. As sfc stabilized and grew as a community, this issue became clearer. During this time, the community gradually recognized that some campers have such extraordinary needs that it limits their ability to give to, never mind participate in, the community as a whole. When they arrive at camp, such individuals abandon their usual coping mechanisms and become vulnerable almost to the point of losing their moorings. Their annual struggle is challenging for them and places a significant strain on the community. Serena's story reflects a composite of camper experiences:

> When I first came to sfc, my husband and I were barely coping with the challenges of our marriage, due in large part to my ongoing struggle with a difficult childhood. After our first year at camp, when I felt like we were the couple from another planet, I began to relax at camp. For a couple of years, both my husband, Jake, and I enjoyed not only camp but being at camp together.
>
> Then, for some reason, soon after Virginia left, I found myself coming to camp and falling apart. I felt like the minute I got on the truck to go down to Pico Blanco, I began to dissolve. By the time we were setting up our tent, I was bawling. While everyone else was greeting people and catching up, I was hiding in my tent sobbing. I would try to do work on what was going on with me, but it felt like no one could help me the way Virginia did, and so I would just get frustrated and unhappy.

Letisha, a camp therapist, remarked:

> Working with Serena was a challenge. She attached herself to Virginia and was both willing and able to do incredible work. But when Virginia left, it seemed that Serena was either unwilling or unable to open herself to working with anyone else. It got to the point that I wondered if camp was not making things harder for Serena. It seemed like each year she came, she would go into this well of self-loathing and sense of betrayal. These feelings often came out through struggles in the community. Serena complained a lot and loudly. She inevitably made the same comments in each feedback session and repeatedly asked to do work on the same issue.

Her needs became so great it was very difficult for the community. Not only was it hard for them to watch her disintegration throughout the week, it was also difficult for the community not to begin to target her as she demanded more and more time. Eventually, people simply did not listen to her concerns. Usually this was because of the way she expressed herself, but for some people, they chose not to listen simply because Serena was the one raising the concerns. The interesting thing is that her concerns were often valid, and when another camper raised the issue, the community would listen.

Serena continued her account:

I think things changed for me once I decided to deal with my marriage. I finally separated from my husband. I went back to school, got a job, and life really came together outside of camp. Nevertheless, each year I was still going to camp and falling apart. I mean, here I was a successful professional, finally able to take care of myself, and then I come to camp and become this blubbering idiot. One year I just decided, "No more." I came to camp by myself, set up my tent, went down and did the greeting thing. I think people were kind of shocked by me that year, especially when I volunteered for the Committee.

Being on the Committee was tough. This was the time of the Big Ducks and the Little Ducks, and I was definitely a Little Duck. Most of the time, people just ignored me. Or, if I did say something, it was discounted. What really got me was the time I made a suggestion, which was ignored as usual until Sondra brought it up later in the day, and then everyone said, "Hey, that's a great idea!" I knew then that I had to confront people. So the next year at camp, I asked to do work about my role in the community.

Letisha said:

Over the years, I had worked with Serena individually at camp. I also helped her get into individual therapy, and it was so gratifying to realize how much progress she was making. I knew what she was achieving outside of camp, but at camp things were much more difficult. Serena really had become a scapegoat for the community. Despite her obvious progress, she was seen as "poor Serena" and for several years, she allowed herself to be just that. But when Serena asked me to be her therapist for a work session about her role in the community, I knew she had really turned a corner. I believe Serena annoyed people because she let herself become very vulnerable and very young while she was at camp. This was necessary for her to go through her healing, but it was a drain on the community energy, especially in group sessions.

Even though it seemed like she was not making progress at camp, Serena really did work on her issues. She also became aware of the role she had taken on in the community. After a lot of hard work both at camp and in therapy during the year, Serena was ready to take her place in the community in the manner she wanted. That work session is one that I will never forget.

The session began with Letisha helping Serena tell the group about the work she wanted to do.

Letisha [*standing in front of the group alongside Serena*]: Serena, you and I have talked about how you want this session to be, correct?

Serena [*nods her head but does not speak*].

Letisha: I believe you wanted to start by addressing the community?

Serena [*taking a deep breath*]: This is a very hard thing for me to do, but I want to take my place in this community, and unless I do this work, I think I will never belong. I know a lot of you are thinking, "Oh, here she goes again about how none of us listen to her and whining about how she doesn't belong." I understand why you are thinking that. I know there have been many years when I have come to camp and been kind of like a leech on the camp's energy.

Letisha [*interrupting gently*]: I want to caution you about taking on the negative voice. You were not a leech. You were a member who had very significant needs.

Serena [*standing taller and speaking in a stronger voice*]: Right. And I understand now that some of those needs were almost larger than the community could hold. It didn't help that I had lots of difficulty asking for what I needed. And I know that when people would try to respond, I pretty much sabotaged all those efforts as well.

But I am at a different point in my life now. I have worked very hard here at camp with Letisha and in my therapy during the year. I understand where my struggles began and how I have coped all these years with the damaged child I carry inside of me. In the last two years, I realized that camp allows me to feel and express feelings that I have to hide the rest of the year. When I come to camp, I seem to be falling apart but really I just had to let that child take over while Serena the adult disappeared.

And then two years ago, I decided not to do that anymore. I came to camp and I stayed present as an adult. For the first time, I wanted to join the community as an adult. And I began to speak up with ideas and concerns I have about how we work as a community. I even joined the Committee so that I could become a stronger voice in that community. But when I did that, I didn't feel that anyone really wanted to see or hear me as Serena the adult.

So I have decided that I want to say to the community that I have changed and I want to be recognized as the adult that I am now, not the wounded person who used to fall apart whenever I came to camp in the past. I want to be able to grow and make mistakes without people judging me with feelings like, "Look out, Serena's about to fall apart" or "Oh no, here she goes again."

Letisha: Is that it? Does that cover what you wanted to say?

Serena: I guess, for now, but I will probably have more.

Letisha [*smiling*]: I'm sure you will, but I would like to take some time now and let people respond to what you have said so far. Let's have people tell you how they feel about what you have said and how they perceive you in the community. And I would like you to listen and take in what they say without having to respond. Okay?

Serena: But———

Letisha: *And* we will also have time for you to join in before we finish. Okay?

Serena: Oh, okay.

Letisha [*turning to the group*]: Is that okay with the group?

People in the group nod and murmur their quiet concurrence. Letisha asks who would like to begin. Only a few hands go up, and the first two people talk. Then many people join a line for the microphone and talk with Serena. These comments are reflective of the group responses:

Alisa: Serena, I'm so glad you are doing this work today. I hope you know how important you are to me and how much the time we spend together means to me. I have worried about you, especially when you went through the divorce. But even when you were struggling, you were my rock, helping me with my struggles and my divorce. I just wish I could have helped you more when things were so hard for you.

Cass: Serena, I have only known you the last two years, but I have really enjoyed our talks, and I have admired your energy and commitment to camp. I have been puzzled when it seems to me that people do not listen to you the same way they listen to others, and I knew there was some history that I didn't understand. I'm glad that you decided to do this work because it helps me know you better. I want you to know that as far as I am concerned, you have and always will have a place in this community.

Paloma: I think I may be one of the people you are talking to. When you talked to us just then, it really helped me become aware of how I have responded to you in the past. I would shut you off when you would be so upset about the same thing year after year.

But I also want you to know that I was glad you decided to join the Committee, because it gave me a chance to get to know you better in a different way. Because of our time together at Committee meetings, I have been able to see the changes you have made. I do value the contributions you make to our discussions here at camp and in the Committee, and I am very glad you did this work today.

Nelson: You and I have had lots of struggles over the years, and I know that I have not always been supportive, as you may have wanted, especially when you decided to leave your husband. But as I see you today and really hear what you are saying, I want you to know how impressed I am with the person you have become. I also feel you are an important person to camp. I want you to let me know if there is anything I do or say that contributes to the feelings you have that you do not belong.

After about another five minutes of comments, Letisha turned to Serena and asked if she wanted to respond.

> Serena: I guess I feel pretty overwhelmed. It's helpful to hear people talk about how they feel and that some of my feelings about how people were responding to me are accurate. Part of that has been hard to hear. At the same time, it is also good to know that people are open to talking about the past and to seeing who I am now. I guess I'm not totally trusting that everyone has been completely honest, but I do think this is a beginning.

> Letisha: And no one expects that this one work session is going to change patterns that have been set over the years. But just like it has taken you a lot of time and a lot of work to make the changes you have made, it will also take time and work for things to change for you here at camp. I think what is important is that the issue has been raised, and you have been able both to tell people how you feel and to also hear how they feel in response.

> Serena: It's important to me that I have also been able to tell people how I have changed. I want people to see that even if I struggle while I am at camp, I am no longer falling apart. I am strong, and I can care for myself, and I do have good ideas and opinions.

> Letisha: I agree. That is probably the strongest message you have given. As I listened to the comments people have shared with you, I believe that they have heard the message as well.

> [*To the group*]: As we end this session, I again want to remind everyone that not everything is changed or fixed. Serena will still have her moments, each of you will have your reactions to those moments, and some of your reactions will be based on both your history as a child and your history with Serena.

> But as the struggles happen, it is important to remember that things have changed. If you find that you are having a reaction to Serena, first check in with yourself and make sure you are not operating on old reactions or things in you that Serena triggers. Then, if you can, share your feelings with Serena and let her know how her reactions are causing you to react.

And Serena, I hope that you will now feel able to go to individuals and check out their reactions if you feel you are not being heard.

Combining a therapeutic program with an intentional community can contribute to both the therapy and the community. The combination can also be fraught with challenges. In the example above, Serena worked through first her individual issues and then her issues with the community. In other cases, the community was not able to support both the person and the behavior. As one camp therapist explained:

> We try to hold both the person and their behavior in this community. Virginia taught that each person has an innate value simply by virtue of being. Therefore, each person in this community has value despite his or her behavior and struggles. But it is a challenge to provide the support to everyone. There have been people who have come to camp and their needs have either been too great or they simply have not been able to fit with the process that happens here at camp. I feel most badly when we are unable to hold such a person in the community. People have left camp hurt and angry, and we have been unable to get them to return and continue to work on the issue at camp.

As an organization, sfc acknowledges that its type of intentional community experience is not appropriate for all families or individuals. The Camp handbook provides a caution regarding the camp's therapeutic services:

> A Word about Therapeutic Services
> Families come to sfc for a variety of reasons. If you are seeking therapy at camp, we suggest that you talk with the camp registrar to be certain that what you need and what occurs at camp is a good fit.

As much as possible, sfc screens potential campers during the application process to make sure that people who come to camp will both benefit from and contribute to the community. As one Committee member said:

> We find the best way to find new members is to have old campers recruit the new campers. Then we know that someone who is part of camp and knows what happens at camp is not only finding someone who "fits" but also is telling the new person what we are all about.

The camp registrar added:

> It is hard to screen people for camp. I have read enough letters
> over the years that I can usually sense if there might be a problem.
> Usually a phone call can clear up any confusion. Because most new
> families are referred by someone from camp, we can check with them
> as well. When we run into problems, it is usually because we have
> made some sort of exception or we need new families and we don't
> take the time we usually take to make sure they are a good fit.

To address problems that had occurred in the past, SFC decided to
use a probationary status for new referrals. The probationary status is
described in the SFC handbook:

> The first year of camp is used by families and by SFC to mutually
> decide if participation in the SFC community is a good fit for the family
> and for the camp. Campers who are invited and choose to return to
> camp for a second year are accepted into the community and invited
> to return each year.

This one-year probationary status helps the community and the
potential members recognize that not all people work well within this
type of community. Although few families have been uninvited, people have self-selected out of the community for many reasons. In
some instances, family circumstances change and the family members
decide to put their energy into other ways to be together. In other
cases, families simply do not feel comfortable in SFC's intense environment. For some parents, the children's commitment helps them overcome their initial discomfort or lack of enthusiasm for camp. As one
long-time camper recounted:

> I found camp so difficult in the beginning. Just being at Pico
> Blanco with young children was so hard, and then I didn't feel
> comfortable with the group. I never felt like I belonged in the
> beginning. But my son loved it, and he just lived to go to camp, so we
> hung in. And now I can't imagine my life without camp!

Who Gets to Go to Camp

Children's commitment to camp and their role in the community
led to a different type of challenge during these middle years. The
community exists to meet the needs of its members, to facilitate their

emotional and psychological growth and, when needed, to protect those who are struggling with psychological problems. One of the most significant events children face early in their lives is divorce. For many of its children and teens, SFC provides a safe and nurturing place to deal with the inevitable pain and upset caused by divorce. For others, the impact of their parents' changing lives threatens the safety they find at camp. The following story illustrates how camp deals with the conflict between parents' needs and children's needs, particularly during a divorce. The following story is based on events that happened at camp. To maintain confidentiality, we have changed names and circumstances.

Shane and Bethany were eleven and twelve, respectively, when their parents divorced. Both children had attended SFC since they were toddlers accompanying their parents, Carmen and Timothy. They are enthusiastic, positive kids who yearned to return to Pico Blanco and the SFC environment each year, as Shane explained:

> Ever since I can remember, I have counted the months all year till we could go back to camp. Most kids live for holidays like Halloween or Christmas, but not me. I was always waiting for that last week in June. When I was little, it was so much fun to go to Pico Blanco and play in the fort and the stream. I liked jumping up and down on the mattresses while the grownups acted all goofy. But as I got older, I began to understand what they were doing in sessions, and I liked to go and learn about families and stuff.
>
> I guess that's why I wasn't too surprised when my parents got divorced. I had watched their work and I understood why it was so hard for them to get along. It really helped that I had my own group to go to for support. The other kids knew what it was like to find out your parents aren't going to live together and how scary it is not to know where you are going to live or anything. Camp was even more important to me after my parents split up.

Bethany concurred:

> I don't know what I would have done without camp those years my parents were falling apart. My mom was crying all the time and my dad was, like, just gone, except when we came to camp. Then we were still a family. We did work together, and Shane and I told our parents how we felt about what was happening to us. In the end, I came to understand that we could still be a family even if we didn't all live together all the time.

But every year at camp, we get to be a whole family. We all stood together and got introduced as a family, and I felt, like, at least for one week a year, I had a regular family like the other kids. And then my dad went and ruined it for all of us.

Several years after his divorce, Timothy entered into a relationship with Nora. Although Nora had developed a superficial relationship with Timothy's children, she did not feel that the children had accepted her relationship with Timothy and wanted to become more involved in activities with the children. Timothy said:

> You know, when I proposed the idea that Nora come to camp, I thought this would be a way for her to join the family. I really misjudged how the kids would react. I was more concerned about how Carmen would feel. I never thought the kids would have a problem. I remember when I told them all about it, the kids stayed quiet and didn't really say anything. Of course, by then it was a done deal.

Carmen related:

> When Timothy told me he wanted to invite Nora to camp, I didn't know how to feel. I was concerned, but I knew he wanted Nora to experience that part of his life. And for me, our relationship was over, so I guess I didn't think it was that big a deal. And the kids didn't seem to really care one way or the other.

The evening after Timothy told his children that he was inviting Nora to camp, Bethany and Shane stayed overnight with friends from SFC, Lisa and Matt. Both Bethany and Shane were angry about their dad's announcement and feeling hopeless about their lack of control over who would go to camp with them that year. When they shared the news about Nora, Lisa told them that the Committee has to approve any new member of Family Camp, so it was not a done deal. Lisa also told them that Bethany and Shane had been at camp longer, so they had the right to write a letter telling the Committee they did not want Nora to come to camp. With Lisa's support, they wrote the following letter.

> Dear Committee,
> Our names are Shane and Bethany F. We have been members of SFC for 9 years. We are writing to tell you that we do not want our dad's girlfriend, Nora, at camp. Nora is not part of our family. She's only been our dad's girlfriend for 7 months.

We do not want her to come to camp because camp is the only time that our family is together. Our mom will not have a good time at camp if Nora is there and we won't either. If our dad wants to have a vacation with Nora, he can go somewhere with her. He should not bring her to the place that has always been just ours.

Because we have been coming to camp for a long time, we hope you will listen to us and not let Nora come to camp.

—Shane and Bethany F.

After writing the letter, Lisa helped Shane and Bethany mail it to the registrar. Neither child told Timothy or Carmen about the letter.

At the November meeting of the Committee, Cecilia, the camp registrar, informed the Committee that she had received a letter from Nora asking to be approved as a camper as well as a support letter from Timothy. Both their letters spoke of the increasing commitment they had to each other and their desire to experience camp as part of that growing commitment. They also indicated that they hoped the time at camp would help Nora grow closer to Bethany and Shane. In his letter, Timothy indicated that he had discussed inviting Nora with Carmen and the children and that they had no objections.

Cecilia then read the letter from Shane and Bethany. In response, a female Committee member thought:

> This was a challenge for me. I really like Shane and Bethany, and I knew they were unhappy with Timothy's decision to enter into a new relationship. But I was also clear that this was their family issue, and I did not see how the Committee could or should do anything but tell the kids to tell their parents how they felt.

A male board member felt:

> I was thrilled that the kids had written the letter. This is what SFC is all about. Here are two kids who step up as members of camp and let us know how they feel and what they want. I felt strongly that we should support them because they are long-standing . . . if young, . . . members of our community.

Morgan, Lisa's dad and a Committee member said:

> I was surprised when I heard the letter. I suspected Lisa was in on it. On the one hand, I was pleased that she knew enough to use the process, but I wished she had talked to me first. I know how hard

the divorce has been on the Bethany and Shane and that they have not told either of their parents how hurt and angry they feel. So I saw the letter more as a way the kids were expressing their feelings about the divorce than their objection to Nora coming to camp. And I wasn't sure that it was the Committee's role to get involved in what really is a family matter.

As the Committee discussed Nora's application and the children's letter, it was divided about how to proceed. People spoke mostly from two positions. On one side, members felt that the Committee should honor the children's desire not to have Nora accepted. On the other side, members felt that the children's parents needed to deal with the children's concerns while the Committee dealt with the application as it would any other.

Those holding the first position focused on the fact that the children were campers who objected to a new person coming into camp. They argued that the Committee should consider children's concerns just as they would consider the objections of any other members. Those on the other side pointed out that the children's concerns were not about whether Nora would be an appropriate member for SFC. Their concerns were about the struggles going on in their family.

Several other members of the Committee remained unaligned and helped focus the discussion on the role of the Committee. Carl, the camp president, commented:

> I think both sides of this issue have valid points. What I do not hear discussed, though, is whether we as a camp really have any role in the issue. It is clear that the children and the parents are not communicating. Timothy writes that the kids have no objections, yet here is their letter. And we don't know how Carmen feels. So maybe the best we can do is take what we know and help the family talk to each other and work this out as a family rather than as a problem for camp to solve.

After much discussion, most members came to the opinion that the Committee should accept Nora's application and help the children communicate directly with their parents about their concerns regarding Nora. One female board member stated:

> It was a difficult discussion for me. Our family had struggled a lot before my children would accept that both my ex-husband and I had moved into new relationships. I empathized with all the different

members of the family, especially the kids. Despite those feelings, I also believed that the Committee should encourage the kids to take these issues to their parents and they, as a family, should deal with how the kids were feeling. The Committee's job was to accept or deny the application, and there was no reason not to accept Nora at camp.

The Committee decided that, in her role as registrar (and therefore the contact person between new applicants and the Committee), Cecilia would contact Bethany and Shane. She would explain that the Committee had accepted Nora's application but was also concerned about their feelings about Nora and wanted to help them work that out within their family. The Committee also instructed Cecilia to offer support—from the Committee or any other member of camp that they chose—to help them talk with their parents.

During the next month, a flurry of e-mails flew among family members and the Executive Committee members, who are responsible for conducting camp business between Committee meetings. After initial resistance by Timothy and the children, a meeting was held among Timothy, Nora, Carmen, Shane, and Bethany. Morgan attended as a representative of the Committee. At the meeting, the family agreed that they all, including Nora, would attend camp that year. They also agreed that they, not including Nora, would work at camp regarding how the children felt about the changes that were occurring in the family and about having Nora at camp.

At the Committee's March meeting, Cecilia and Morgan reported on the activities and final resolution. The Committee again processed the issues related to its decision and reached consensus that the Committee can provide support to all members of a family but that problems among children and parents need to be resolved at the family rather than the community level.

Community Implications

Starting in 1993 and continuing over the next few years, SFC moved through the stage of Redefinition. Beginning with the struggle to redefine the roles and behaviors at Family Camp between men and women, the energy expressed was what the Satir Change Model called Integration. This energy focuses on analyzing new patterns and defining new terms and conditions.

Family Camp emerged from this period of Redefinition with a new structure of leadership, new expectations, boundaries around male and female relationships, greater equity in meeting the needs of the entire community, and new expectations regarding individual behavior and group compliance. Through this Redefinition, sfc moved successfully to Synergy, the next stage of community development.

In Synergy, a community utilizes the new definitions and structure created in the Redefinition stage to achieve greater goals for the community as a whole. The energy of Implementation fuels this Synergy stage. This energy focuses on using the new structure and finding a comfortable new balance within the system.

The Camp Nag, ad hoc groups, and the development of policies are all examples of how sfc shifted camp functions to a higher level of organization. Camp settled into a "new normal" or comfort zone that represented a balance in which camps was meeting the needs of the majority effectively.

6

Ennui

The ten annual camps held between 1993 and early 2003 span the community's development through the stages of Redefinition and Synergy, ending with movement toward Ennui. By the year 2003, SFC had grown into a community that was both stable and stagnant. Camp evaluations indicated that the program was predictable and a bit boring. Although the community was not looking for problems, it was apparent that it had fallen into a rut. The Committee recognized that SFC depended almost entirely on senior members of the community and lacked adequate connection with the youth, who represented SFC's future.

These realities came together to create a new status quo. Camp moved toward the final stage of community development, Ennui. Due largely to the group's structural success and meeting the majority's needs, abundant energy was available to focus on personal growth. This growth led to having more time and inclination to question the status quo and debate new directions in which to take the community.

At the beginning of the twenty-first century, Nelson and Phyllis looked back on almost twenty-five years of attending SFC. Over the years, they have brought two more children into the world and raised all three to adulthood successfully. Nelson reflected:

> Camp has been a major part of our family life. We plan our
> summers around the last week in June. There was one year when our
> youngest, Jordan, was ten and ended up in the hospital the day before
> we were to leave for camp. He had appendicitis and needed
> emergency surgery, which was terrifying for Phyllis and me, but in the

end worked out fine. Of course, we canceled camp. We just didn't see how we could take him from the hospital to Pico Blanco. Jordan, on the other hand, was determined to go and in the end he won out. Jordan told his doctor all about camp and how much he wanted to be there. After listening to Jordan and finding out that there was a pediatrician at camp, the doctor agreed to let Jordan go. We got there two days late, and Jordan was received like a returning hero!

Camp has changed for us now. All three kids are grown and on their own. At this point, only Jordan continues to come to camp and that's not every year. He, his partner, and her son come to camp as often as they can. I'm disappointed that Mia isn't more involved. I always thought she would be the one to come as an adult. She came when she was single, but after she got married, things changed. Duane, her husband, tried camp for a year or maybe two, but it was not for him. I think coming to camp as a couple is especially hard when one of the couple grew up as part of the camp family. Talk about having a lot of in-laws around! In the end, I just don't think Duane could tolerate the intensity of the relationships we all have with each other. The fact that he doesn't like camping didn't help, either.

So we are adjusting to an empty nest at home as well as at camp. One year, Phyllis and I came without any kids. Being alone in the tent is fine. As soon as the kids became teenagers, they went off on their own, and we have always enjoyed having that space to ourselves. But when we are at dinner or the kids are playing volleyball or ping pong, I find myself looking around for one of mine. Camp was the time when we reconnected as a family. We all lead very busy lives during the year, and we used our week at camp to be together on a deeper, more meaningful level. The kids would talk about their lives, about their struggles, about their future. We all went to sessions, and certainly Phyllis and I did a lot of work at camp. The kids had the teen group and then the young adult group, but we also talked and shared just as a family, and I miss that a lot.

Many of the families who came to camp with young kids during the Pico Blanco time are going through the same thing. Phyllis and I talk with Carl and Sherry a lot. They have the same situation with their son-in-law as we have with Duane. In many ways, I miss seeing Julia and Joey almost as much as I miss seeing my own kids. Right now, these kids are starting their adult lives, and it is just hard for them to fit in camp as well. We hope that will change, especially when they become parents, and that they will return to camp and take over as leaders.

Camp has changed a lot since those early years at Pico Blanco. We are kind of becoming a graying organization. Right after we moved to Camp Loma, we had an influx of new families with young kids, but even those kids are in their teens, and some are young adults. We don't get new families every year because we are at capacity when we have about eighty families, and since most of our families come back each year, there is not a lot of room for growth. It is raising some interesting issues for the future of camp.

Phyllis shared her perspective:

> I have changed so much over the years and feel so at peace with myself and my life, and I know that's because of my experience at camp. In many ways, I grew up at camp. Now that my kids are on their own, I can focus on me and my life and what I want to do now that my role of mother had changed from full-time mom to being a support person when my kids decide they need one. I had my kids young, so I have a lot of my life ahead of me, and I want to make that time meaningful for me. My experience at camp helped me decide what I wanted to do with the rest of my life and helped me have the courage to go do it. I think I am an example of what it means to become "fully human." My experiences at camp have helped me not only understand but also accept my early life and all that happened. I have been able to accept the child that was so rejected and unwanted and to nurture her and care for her. Each year that I came to camp, I learned more about my needs and how to care for myself. I was finally able to move from being the caretaker of everyone else to being my own caretaker.
>
> Once I made that switch, things got so much better in my relationships, not just with Nelson and the kids but with my friends and then with the world around me. I made some important decisions about my future. I went back to school and got my license as a nurse and then as a nurse practitioner. Now I work with terminally ill children and their families. It is hard, painful work but so important, and I know that my skills and life experiences are being used to their fullest.
>
> I could never have reached this place without camp. Not only what I learned at camp but the support and caring that I have received. I finally found a true family that not only helped me heal my wounds but also gave me the support to live my life to the fullest.

In 2005, SFC celebrated its twenty-fifth year of operation, dating from the first camp at Pico Blanco, in 1980. During those twenty-five years, the community grew from Virginia's experiment into a mature community made up of individuals and families who return year after year to participate in a magical week-long experience of challenge and nurturance of each person as well as the community as a whole. The camp has also slowly moved to the stage of Ennui. In this stage, a community enjoys the fruits of earlier developmental stages and identifies new challenges. At sfc, this occurred because of the successes of the new structure, the rededicated Committee leadership, and the different roles and rules defined during the middle years.

Satir Family Camp Organization

At twenty-five years, the community continues to comprise three major parts: the annual camp, the Committee, and the therapeutic team. A fourth piece is the Pulse of the Camp committee.

The Annual Camp

sfc continues to meet during the last week of June each year. Attendees are individuals and families who have applied to and been accepted by the Committee. The Committee accepts up to 135 people. To provide services to this population, it contracts with a cook, a cook's assistant, and a seven-person team of therapists. In 2005, 110 people attended, ranging in age from 2 to 92 years. The vast majority of campers have attended camp at least twice. One couple has attended since the first camp started by Jackie Schwartz in 1977.

The Committee

The Committee continues to be the camp's governing body. It is responsible for governance between the annual camps and authorizes the Executive Committee to handle camp business between the Committee's quarterly meetings. The Executive Committee also handles confidential issues involving camp participants, at camp and during the rest of the year. Currently, the Executive Committee comprises the president, president-elect, vice-president, secretary, treasurer, registrar, past president, and therapists' liaison.

The Therapeutic Team

At the time of this writing, sfc contracts with a team of seven therapists to provide therapeutic services both at camp and, on request, to individuals and groups (such as the Committee) during the year. The team includes both male and female therapists, all of whom are licensed or trained in Satir methods, or both. The decision to contract with licensed therapists only or therapists working under the supervision of a licensed therapist has been a recent change at sFC. It reflects the increased awareness of the camp's and Committee's exposure to liability lawsuits as well as California state law regarding who can provide therapeutic services. It signals how the field of mental health has changed. Like many therapists in the 1970s and '80s, Virginia Satir was not a licensed therapist.

Changes in state law also changed how the camp responds to issues of child abuse at camp or within its population. When Virginia first began practice in the late 1950s, child abuse, particularly child sexual abuse, was an unspoken secret generally kept within the family. Virginia provided services to many clients referred by the then young and developing field of child protective services. People who attended camp during the Virginia years often brought with them histories of child abuse. Yet, even by the mid-1980s, when Virginia left camp, sFC had no specific policy regarding child abuse or its reporting.

By 1990, California law mandated that mental health practitioners who have knowledge or reasonable suspicion of a child at risk of or being abused must report that knowledge or suspicion to a child protection agency. Because mental health practitioners both attend and provide services at camp, the Committee designates a licensed therapist at each camp to report any case of child abuse that becomes known, occurs, or is suspected while families are at camp. At the beginning of each camp, someone informs campers of all mental health reporting requirements and introduces the therapist responsible for reporting.

During camp nowadays, different members of the therapeutic team work with adults, young adults, teens, and children. Whenever possible, at least one member of the team attends all group meetings. The therapists also meet with individuals, families, and small groups.

For most of sFC's middle years, five therapists worked at camp. The intensity of the job, along with therapists' health problems, led to the decision to recruit additional members for the therapeutic team. Laura Dodson recruited additional therapists, who in turn have recruited others. New therapists have attended camp for one year as interns. Working a year as an intern gives the camp and the therapist an opportunity to meet and work together prior to making an ongoing commitment.

The community and the Committee, in particular, use the terms *facilitator* and *therapist* interchangeably. These reflect the two roles that therapists now perform at camp. The team's primary task at camp continues to be in the role of therapists. In addition, the therapeutic team also works in partnership with the community and the Committee to facilitate and enhance community growth. At times, combining these two roles has been a challenge for the therapeutic team as well as for the camp.

Pulse of the Camp Committee

During the middle years, the Executive Committee began to meet daily at camp with the therapists to deal with problems or concerns that arose. Informally, they called these meetings the "Pulse of the Camp committee." As things stabilized during the late middle years, the Camp Committee, with the therapists' support, examined the role of the Pulse Committee and how it fit with the role of the sfc Committee. Originally, the Pulse Committee made both governance and therapeutic decisions at camp. After some campers raised issues about that, the Executives and the Committee as a whole agreed that the Pulse Committee needed to take its governance decisions to the whole Committee for a final decision. As a result, rather than being an extension of the Executive Committee, the newly defined Pulse Committee would be representative of the entire community and would exist only for the week of camp. That committee's purpose continued to be to deal proactively with any problems or concerns that arose during camp.

Representatives from all groups in camp now participate on the Pulse Committee. Members include a representative of the teen and young adult groups as well as a member from the camp as a whole. The camp president and the entire therapeutic team also participate. In the sfc tradition, people volunteer to be members of the Pulse Committee. If more than one person from each group volunteers, the names are put in a hat and one name is drawn. During camp, the Pulse Committee meets each morning and discusses any and all issues affecting camp. A member of the Pulse Committee may raise an issue or issues may be brought to the Pulse Committee by anyone in the community. The Pulse Committee is yet another iteration that the sfc uses to address community as well as individual and family issues.

Revitalizing the Camp Experience

From 2000 to 2004, sfc settled into a comfortable routine of camps that were organized around group sessions and family events. By 2004, camp seemed to recreate the same program year to year. The five (and eventually seven) therapists worked well with each other, and campers knew them well. In most cases, work sessions during those years focused on campers who came to camp with self-identified issues that they wanted to address during camp. In fact, so many people came to camp to work that the therapists usually had all work sessions committed to individuals by the beginning of the week.

During the same time, the special-interest groups, such as the women's group and the men's group, grew in importance as more people chose to do therapeutic work in the smaller settings. A growing number of campers gradually saw their affiliation to these groups as being their primary connection to the community. By 2004, the established affinity groups included those for men, women, elders, young adults, teens, and children.

In the same way that the therapy program became routine, the community activities also became predictable. Each year featured Family Games, Free University, Party Night, Skit Night; Family Bingo, a community-wide game to introduce people to each other; and the auction, to raise money for camp.

After four years of relatively predictable camps, the evaluations that campers filled out showed that they were becoming bored with camp. They also expressed concern that the community was dividing into special-interest groups, leaving little free time simply to relax and renew old or establish new friendships.

After receiving this feedback, the Committee took specific steps to address these concerns. When a community event became stale, they dropped it from the next year's program. They created new activities to help address divisions within the community. During the first lunch at the 2005 camp, leaders asked campers to sit at assigned tables. Each table included members from the different age groups within camp including seniors, adults, young adults, teens, and children, as well as new campers and experienced campers. During lunch, each group had the same list of questions to guide conversation about their interest in and hopes for camp, both then and in the future. Each group had a recorder who wrote up and posted the group's responses to the questions. During the week, the therapists also used the responses to enrich discussion at Temperature Reading and during all the group sessions.

The Pulse Committee also identifies individual family concerns and issues or concerns that involve the community. Just as family work sessions help generate discussion within families, it helps bring to the surface community issues, particularly issues about the way the community operates and organizes itself.

One significant issue during this period is the way sfc balances the needs of its individual members with the needs of the community. The following story illustrates how complicated this issue can be in a therapeutic community. It began on the opening day of camp, when the Executive Committee told a camper to leave. This highly unusual incident demonstrates the potential strain between a family's need for confidentiality and the community's need to process such a critical event. While we based this version on events at sfc, we have changed the names and some of the circumstances to protect confidentiality.

Whose Needs Take Priority?

The Executive Committee told Nicole, age 22, to leave camp after Nicole's mother, Celeste, informed the Executive Committee that Nicole had brought marijuana to camp, that her mother saw her smoking it while at camp, and that Nicole (on probation for drug charges) was violating the terms of her probation. The Executive Committee also knew that Nicole had smoked marijuana at camp before and that she had agreed in the young adult group that if she smoked at camp in the future, she would be told to leave camp.

The Executive Committee met with Nicole, who admitted having and using marijuana and agreed to leave camp at once. That committee also met with and informed Celeste of its decision to have Nicole leave camp. After those two meetings, Executive Committee members shifted their concern to informing the community that they had asked a camper to leave. The Executive Committee and the therapists agreed that Eliana, as therapist, and Paul, as camp president, would address the issue at the first Temperature Reading. To honor confidentiality and because Celeste had asked for time to talk with other members of her family, it was agreed not to share the story about why and what led up to the decision with the community.

Almost everyone was at that Temperature Reading, and the mood was optimistic and jovial. As the agenda moved to "Announcements," Eliana and Paul joined the line of campers waiting to speak. They faced the group knowing that this announcement would have a huge impact on this year's camp.

> Eliana: I have a difficult announcement to make. This morning, the Executive Committee and therapists asked a camper to leave camp. Because of problems that we did not become aware of until after camp began, we felt this individual

could not remain at camp. I know many of you will have questions about this. I am also sure that you can understand what a difficult time this is for the family involved. We want to assure you that we are offering all of them support and, in the spirit of that support, we want to maintain their confidentiality.

Paul: I don't have a lot to add to what Eliana just said, except that it was a difficult decision, and right now we are doing everything we can to help the family.

Fred [*speaking from the amphitheater*]: Does that mean that the rest of the family is staying at camp?

Paul: As far as we know. Listen, we don't want to take up more time right now, so if any of you have more questions or concerns, how about you meet with me after Temperature Reading?

Although the process at Temperature Reading continued, most people were distracted as they tried to take in the meaning of Paul and Eliana's announcement. Many of the adults begin talking among themselves, and the group's tone changes from concern to displeasure and finally anger. Temperature Reading ends quickly, and a group of seven people quickly stand in a circle around Paul. Most are members of the Committee and immediately express their dismay at not being involved in the decision.

Sissy: Paul, how could you make a decision like that without talking to the whole Committee?

Fred: I sure want to know the same thing. This is the first time that I have ever heard of someone being asked to leave camp. I assume you had good reasons, but I really have problems with the process.

[*More people begin talking at once, most agreeing with the previous comments.*]

Paul: Okay, okay. Obviously, people are upset. I want you to know it was an upsetting thing to have to do. Right now, all I can do is ask you to trust the Execs on this one. There just was not time to pull everyone together and go through all the information. Heck, we were still getting information as we made the decision.

Sissy: That's exactly my point. Here go the Execs again, making really critical decisions without taking the time to think through the implications———

Paul:Now, wait a minute, you know we thought———

Sissy: Please, let me finish. *You* may feel you thought it through, but what about how the rest of camp feels? While I was coming up to talk to you, I heard one of the new campers say she hopes there isn't something she did that would cause her to get thrown out. So I stopped and assured her that we don't do that here, but then she looked at me— "Hello, it just happened"—and I felt like an idiot.

Fred: So what did you say to her?

Sissy: I told her we had never done it before, and I was sure there had to be a really serious reason that caused it to happen, and that I was going to find out. [*She turns back to Paul and asks*]: So what did happen, Paul?

Paul: All I can say right now is that it was very serious and required the action we took. I just can't go into the details until we know that the family has all the information. As soon as we know the family knows what is going on, then we'll get together and decide how to handle the fallout from this.

James: I guess I'm willing to wait a bit, but I don't want to see something as important as this hidden behind confidentiality. This is just why I joined the Committee, to prevent a small group from making all the decisions for the entire camp. If Virginia had been here, we would have just taken the whole thing to Temperature Reading and then there wouldn't be all these paranoid vibes going around.

Carl: Now, wait a minute, James, you know as well as I do that if this happened when Virginia was here, she would have just made the decision herself and no one would have known, or if they did, we sure wouldn't have asked about it!

James [*defensively*]: That wasn't always true.

Paul [*obviously irritated*]: Look, I just don't have the time to debate what Virginia would or would not have done. I need to go talk with Eliana and Glen about the work session and let them know what people are saying. Sissy, I appreciate the feedback, and I will make sure the facilitators know. I promise we will have a full Committee discussion as soon as things are a little clearer.

With that, the group broke up. Most people went to get their chairs and stop for coffee before the first work session began. Paul met with the Executive Committee and facilitators, who had taken seats at a picnic table away from the dining area. As they talked, the Executive Committee and the rest of the therapists expressed a sense of relief. Nicole had left without a fuss, and the announcement to the camp had not created a crisis.

Paul was less comfortable. He expressed his concern that the community's initial reaction might not remain benign. He told the group about his impromptu meeting after Temperature Reading.

> Paul: At this point, people seem most upset about the process, and no one is pushing for the actual information about why we asked Nicole to leave.
>
> Maura: And it needs to stay that way. We really need to keep the family's confidentiality. I don't think Celeste has talked to the rest of the family yet. Besides, this just isn't something everyone needs to know about.
>
> Paul [*speaking over others who begin to talk*]: Listen, I think we have the potential for a big problem. Here we are with a significant reason for asking Nicole to leave, which we can't explain to camp. I mean it about people not really accepting what we said this morning. Sissy is already pushing hard for why the decision was made so quickly without any other input and, of course, James is focusing on the past—you know, "If this had happened when Virginia was here. . . ."

Groans break out among the group, and several make side comments about Sissy and James.

> Maura: Wait a minute, I know some people annoy us, but their reaction is usually an indicator of how others in camp are feeling, so let's think this thing through. The opening work session starts in about fifteen minutes. I think we will get a better sense of what is going on there. How about we begin the session by letting people to talk about their reactions? Not

to ask questions about the details but to say how they are feeling about the fact that a camper was asked to leave.

Glen: Would it be okay if I start the Session? I was not part of the announcement, so it may be easier for me to keep the focus on people's feelings rather than on the details of why it happened. I also think it will be important to keep the focus off Eliana for a bit. You know how some of the older campers still tend to identify her with Virginia. We want to be clear this was not a decision that was made arbitrarily or just by Eliana.

The group agrees and heads out to join the majority of adult campers, who have convened at the session area. As agreed, Glen begins the session.

Glen: We want to welcome you all to our first work session. We use this session to discuss our hopes and wishes for the week. Before we begin that process, I want to acknowledge that the announcement about a camper being asked to leave camp has been difficult for people. I know there is confusion about what happened and why. We want to give each of you an opportunity to talk about your reactions. As we do with reactions at a work session, we ask that you focus on how this decision affects you and your feelings about camp. [*Motioning toward the therapists, who are sitting to the side of the group, he continues*]: None of us or members of the Executive Committee is in a position to discuss the specific reasons that led to this decision. Those issues are confidential, and because members of the family remain in camp, we ask that you respect their right to privacy. However, we do want to know how you are feeling and what concerns this decision brings up for you.

Alisa: I'll start. The fact that someone can be told to leave makes me uncomfortable. I mean, what if I do something and then I'm asked to leave? It just makes me feel really unsafe. [*She passes the microphone to the next speaker.*]

Patrice: I'm a new camper, and I felt so good last night. This seemed like such a welcoming, friendly group; and now that has changed for me. People seem upset and so unclear.

It's like no one really knows what's going on, and that is making me feel unsure about how safe I feel here.

Nelson: I'm a member of the Execs, so I was in on the decision. I support the decision and want all of you to know that although it was made quickly, it was not made without thought and consideration for the individual, for the family, and for the camp. I also know that the process was less than what we want and strive for here at camp. I hope at some point this week we can take a look at the process and decide if we need to do something that would make it work better in the future.

James: I joined the Committee this year to try and show that I can do more than just complain. But now, just as camp starts, we have the same problem happening. We do not have the opportunity to address these issues as a community. Instead, a small group of people gets together, makes significant decisions, and then insists that only they can know the reasons for those decisions. Maybe there are confidentiality issues here, but somehow when something this big happens, we have to do better to make sure that the whole community gets to process the issue. I mean, come on, we just told someone to leave our community!

Maura: That's true, James, but I was also involved in the decision, and I can assure you it was not made lightly or impulsively. We are trying to do our best to address a huge community issue in a way that also protects the rights of the individuals involved.

Sean: Well, I think you were impulsive. Why couldn't this have been addressed by more than just the Execs and when more time could have been taken to think things through?

Glen: I think we have two discussions happening here. One is the process of how the decision was made, and the other is about how people are feeling. I realize it may be difficult to keep these two separate, but I want to be sure that we address people's feelings and then we can figure out how to address the process issues.

Sissy: Well, I'm not sure they can be separated, but I will tell you how I'm feeling. I just feel angry and somewhat betrayed. I asked my sister to come this year and spent all this time telling her about how wonderful the community is because we process everything and have such a deep sense of trust with each other, and now this happens. [*Looking at her sister, who is sitting beside her*]: I just want you to know that this has never happened before, and I am so sorry.

Brittany [*Sissy's sister*]: I guess I feel confused. I mean, I do not know what's happening and, to tell you the truth, I'm okay with that. I figure you have officers who are responsible for camp and they need to make these decisions. I guess I'm glad that they told us, but in some ways it might have been better if the whole thing had just been kept private.

Maddy: I kind of agree with her. Sorry, I don't know your name. Oh, Brittany. Yeah, I agree with Brittany. This is becoming another big camp drama. Like this will be the "Year We Threw the Camper Out," and I really don't like that. Okay, something happened, a decision was made, and now it's over. I just want to have camp, not spend all week talking about who made the decision and why and all that stuff.

Additional people speak of their discomfort and lack of trust for the group, while others speak in support of the Executive Committee's right to make such a decision. Finally, Nelson gets up to speak again.

Nelson: I agree with what Maddy said a while ago. I also hope this won't become the theme for the week. But at the same time, it is a really big deal for camp to tell someone to leave. I think we need to have a way to make sure that more than just the Execs and the therapists understand what happened so we don't have people talking and guessing all week.

Glen: Well, this seems like a governance issue, which means it should be addressed by the body that is responsible for governance, which is the Committee. Would it work to have the Committee meet and discuss ways to keep the community informed when the Executives make this type of decision and then bring their recommendations and discussion to the whole camp?

At this point, the group seemed to reach a consensus: to have the Committee handle the issue. The group was then willing to move on to address their "Hopes and Wishes" for the rest of camp.

Later that day, the young adult group discusses the same issue at its first meeting. Nicole is identified by virtue of her absence, as she has been an active member of that group.

> Megan [*looking around the group*]: Okay, so you know that Nicole is the camper who was asked to leave and that is what all this shit is about, right?

Some of the nine campers nodded in agreement, while several others obviously had not been aware that Nicole is the person who was told to leave. Lincoln and Nita, the two members of the therapist team who attend the young adults group, look concerned. When Nita began to speak, Megan cut her off.

> Megan: Look, I know there is all this stuff about how confidential everything is supposed to be, but I talked with Nicole while she was packing, and she asked me to tell the group what happened. We always share with each other, so I think we have a right to talk about this. [*The group expresses first upset and then anger*].
>
> Lincoln: Okay, we know this is an important issue for the group. Let's just restate that everything we discuss here is confidential unless a group member agrees to have something discussed outside the group. Nicole has asked that what happened to her be discussed here, so she has given us permission to discuss it, but what we talk about needs to stay here, agreed?
>
> Megan: So, when the shit hit the fan, Nicole came to me and we talked. You know she's been struggling with drugs and stuff ever since high school. I kept in touch with her all this year, and she seemed to be doing really good. She's kept her job and her apartment and stayed in N.A. [Narcotics Anonymous]. She's been seeing her mom on and off, and she was really looking forward to camp.

Nicole had been a member of SFC since she was seven, and most of the group was aware of her conflict with her stepfather, Stan.

During that time, the young adults group provided Nicole support both at camp and often throughout the year, particularly as she tried to deal with her increasing substance abuse.

Megan: See, Nicole's mom told her that Stan wasn't coming to camp this year, so Nicole was looking forward to having this time with her mom, you know, just the two of them. Then Stan announces, "Of course I'm coming to camp" and Nicole's mom, just like always, makes nice and tells Nicole to be quiet.

So they come here and get introduced last night as this happy family and afterwards Nicole lost it. She was just so upset that she felt she had to have something to help her get through this week . . . and she smoked some weed. And yeah, she brought some to camp, but she didn't use it on the camp grounds. She went down the road and lit up.

Then, if you can believe it, Nicole's mom shows up and sees her smoking and just goes ballistic. Not only that, but then her mom goes and tells the Executive Committee! So, of course, you know Nicole is just fucked.

Nita [*softly*]: There are other issues about Nicole smoking that joint that made Celeste so concerned.

Megan [*in an annoyed tone*]: You mean her being on probation? Well, okay, there is that. See, Nicole got busted last year and put into a drug diversion program and they make a big deal about No More Drugs. And of course, her mother and Stan totally freaked out last night. So they all did this tough love thing and told Nicole she had to leave camp.

Anyway, Nicole called her dad, and he told her to come and stay with him. And I don't know what they are going to do about her probation stuff.

Nat: Well, isn't that all confidential? We are a camp that helps people, not snitches on them, right? I mean, I thought that's why people come to camp, to get supported and all that shit.

Lincoln [*quietly*]: That is what we try to do, Nat, and it is what we did for Nicole the other two times she brought dope to camp. The first time we knew Nicole was using, we talked with her and helped her get into a program, and she agreed that she would not use at camp.

Then, when she had a relapse last year, we made another agreement with her, but we also told her that if there were any further relapses here at camp, she would be asked to leave. We made that agreement here, right?

Brandon: Well, yeah, you made it, but I don't think we all agreed with it. It was more like, go along with it or she gets kicked out right now, is what I remember.

Janet: That's not exactly the way I remember it, Brandon. I think we were trying to support Nicole staying in treatment. Come on, even Nicole agreed she needed to have some limits to help her stop. So what happens about her probation?

Nita: That's up to Nicole. We will maintain her confidentiality, but we also want to support her dealing with her drug use. So we encouraged her to be honest with her probation office and to explore whether she needs a different kind of treatment. And we held to the consequences we agreed to last year.

Janet: Isn't it true that there could be consequences for all of us because of this? I mean, isn't that why the Committee set up the drug and alcohol policy, to make sure that the camp doesn't get kicked out of here?

Brandon: Yeah, the Committee has that policy, but you know lots of people do drugs at camp and they aren't all just teens and us. Some of them are parents. And let's get real about the great alcohol and drug policy. It says only beer and wine, but my parents have their little supply of gin and tonics in their tent and that cocktail hour is getting longer and longer.

Nita: Yes, drugs at camp put the camp at risk, and that is why the Executive Committee got involved. But I think there are deeper issues here for us to talk about. Nicole is an important part of this group, and she is gone, and I'm wondering how that makes each of you feel?

Rita: Well, I'm probably the newest person here, and I only met Nicole last year, but it makes me feel sad. I wonder what's going to happen to her and how we can help her. And then I think about her mother and her grandparents and wonder how they are doing.

Jules: Yeah, and there's the wonderful camp gossip mill. You just know this is going to be the hot topic for the rest of the week. There'll be all these battles about who made the decision and how [*in a sotto voice*]: "If Virginia were here, we would all talk about it." Man, I can just see how Temperature Reading is going to go for the rest of the week.

Lincoln: Well, I can tell you that this morning, Eliana talked with Nicole. She has gone to stay with her dad and has agreed to tell her probation officer what happened. We have told her that we support her staying in treatment. And if Nicole wants us to, we will also talk to her probation officer.

Brandon: Well, great, the facilitators [therapists] support her, but what about her parents? I bet her stepfather would love to see her go to jail.

Mandy: I'm wondering how Mathew and Marie [Nicole's grandparents] are doing with all of this. I know that was another reason why Nicole wanted to come, 'cause her grandparents finally decided to come back to camp. Course, it also really sucks that this happens just when they come back.

Nicole is the third generation of campers in her family. Several years after her paternal grandparents started to attend camp, they invited her biological father, Don, his wife Celeste, and Nicole (then age 7) to come to camp. Relationships at camp became complicated for the family, as well as for camp, when Nicole's parents divorced several years later. The divorce came after Celeste became involved with Stan, whom she met at Family Camp. This was the first year that Mathew and Marie returned to camp since Celeste and Don were divorced. Don has not returned.

Brandon: Oh yeah, I forgot they're back. Man, is that going to add to the drama. I just hate it when camp gets like this.

Nita: Like what?

Brandon: [*in anger*]: Oh, come on, you know exactly what I mean. There is all this family drama and nobody has any privacy. Look what everyone did when Nicole's mom left her dad. They all took sides and Nicole was miserable for, like, three summers.

Lincoln: And how was it for you, Brandon? As I remember, you
were really close to Don.

Brandon: Well, what do you think? It just sucked. Of course, I
was worried about Nicole, and I really felt bad for Don, too,
but I also thought it was just their business and we all
should have butted out. Instead ———— [*He stops, his head
down and his fists clenched*].

Lincoln [*gently, leaning forward toward Brandon*]: Instead?

Brandon [*loudly*]: Instead, this stupid camp just gossiped away
and then Don left and he never has come back!

Lincoln [*softly*]: Which was hard for you, wasn't it?

Brandon [*with tears in his voice*]: Not as hard as for Nicole, but
yeah, I miss him. He was the closest thing I ever had for a dad
and that asshole Stan went and just ruined it. For all of us.

Mandy [*moving to put her arms around Brandon*]: I miss Don, too.
He was always so much fun. Remember when he put up
the rope swing for us? And he was always hanging out at
the fire pit. I remember the first time I went there at night.
I think I was about ten, and I snuck out of the tent after
my parents were asleep. I came to the edge of the fire and
just kind of stood there. It was Don who invited me to sit
down. He just treated me like one of the teens. I felt like I
was finally part of the really cool group at camp.

Janet: I hate it when stuff like this goes down at camp. It just
ruins the week. I know Nicole has her problems, but I
don't see why what she does has to ruin it for the rest of
us. I was really hoping this would just be a mellow camp.

During the week, the Executives and therapists continue to
balance the needs of Nicole's family with the expectation that the
Committee would process the Executive Committee and therapists'
decision. The second time Eliana called to check on Nicole, she
learned that Nicole had voluntarily entered residential treatment as
an alternative to having her probation revoked.

Knowing that Nicole was cared for, the therapists put their energy
into helping Celeste, who seemed overwhelmed both by what had
happened and by having to tell her former in-laws. As it turned out,
Celeste had not told Mathew and Marie the real reason that the Executive Committee had told Nicole to leave camp. Instead, she told them

that the reasons were private and gave the impression that Nicole had become too upset to be at camp. It was not until Tuesday night, when the grandparents asked Eliana if Nicole was going to be okay, that Eliana realized that the grandparents still did not know why Nicole had left.

At the Wednesday meeting of the Executives and therapists, Eliana continued to advise against a Committee meeting until Celeste told the grandparents the whole story. This did not happen until Thursday morning. By that time, camp was coming to an end, and neither the Committee nor the community had processed the issue. Instead, information was shared among individuals. The young adult group had heard the details at its meeting, and both Celeste and Stan had shared the story with their closest friends. Finally, on Thursday, with Eliana's assistance, Celeste also told Mathew and Marie about Nicole's behavior. By Friday, almost everyone on the Committee knew who had been asked to leave as well as the reasons why.

Each Friday at camp, the Committee holds an open meeting for anyone interested in learning about the Committee. That meeting's agenda focuses on what must be done to close camp. With few exceptions, issues that require discussion are put over to the annual November business meeting. At this particular Friday meeting, Paul recommended and the Committee agreed to table any discussion of the Executive Committee's authority to tell a camper to leave camp. Even Sissy and James agreed that the discussion would be better handled in November.

This decision is typical in that the Committee rarely, if ever, includes the community in discussions of most problems that involve family privacy. In this case, the Committee was particularly reluctant to discuss the matter because Mathew and Marie—founding members of the Committee—had decided to rejoin the Committee and attended the Friday meeting. So did Celeste, who also was a member of the Committee. Their presence pretty well guaranteed that the Committee would delay the discussion until November.

Although things ended quietly for the camp at large, Nicole's family continued struggling up to the very last moment of camp. Mathew and Marie were angry that many campers had learned the real reason for Nicole's departure before they knew. Despite Eliana and Maura's efforts to help mend the rift in the family, Mathew and Marie left camp angry, and Celeste left feeling unsupported, believing that many saw her decision to inform the Committee as more proof that she does not support Nicole.

Between camp's end and the November meeting, Mathew and Marie sent several e-mails to members of the Executive Committee, expressing their upset at how things were handled at camp. In addition, Stan sent several angry e-mails about what he perceived as lack of support for Celeste. After the Executive Committee received these e-mails, copies quickly circulated among the Committee as a whole. Not surprisingly, when the Committee met in November, a sense of discomfort pervaded the group. Celeste, Mathew, and Marie were present, and the tension among them was palpable. As is traditional, the Committee meeting began with check in, a time for members to provide updates of their activities and their families. Seated in a circle, people share events in their lives and the lives of their children. People took turns, and then it was Mathew's time to check in.

> Mathew: Well I'm happy to tell you that Nicole is doing great. After she left camp, she went to stay with Don, and he helped her go to her probation officer and report her violation. The probation officer was supportive, thank god, and Nicole was placed in a three-month in-patient program. Now she just came home and is still living with Don. She goes to an outpatient group. Don goes with her to the family group, and they both seem to be doing okay.
>
> [*Turning to look at Marie, seated next to him*]: Now, if we can just get some closure about how this was handled at camp, I think things will be good.

> Marie: I agree things are better for all of us. Nicole is looking for work, and she comes to visit us almost every week. It's so nice to have the family together. I will say though, I still have a lot of feelings about what happened at camp, but at least things worked out for Nicole.

While Mathew and Marie spoke, Celeste sat across the room, first with a pained and then an angry expression. She clutched the hand of the woman next to her and, by the end of Marie's statement, was in tears. The sharing continued around the circle until it was Celeste's turn.

> Celeste: Well, things are not so great for me. I don't see much of Nicole any more. She refuses to come to the house if Stan is there. It feels like I'm in the middle of this huge mess and there is no way out for me. I'm really glad Nicole is

doing better, and I try to see her when I can after work, but it's hard. I know everybody is mad at me because I reported her probation status to the Committee, but I just didn't know what else to do.

At this point, Celeste began crying and was too upset to talk. She rushed out of the room. Paul suggested a break. After time for coffee and cooling of emotions, Paul reconvened the meeting.

Paul: I think we have two things we need to deal with about the past camp. There are still feelings about what happened to Nicole and her family during camp. And we need to process the decision itself. I'd like to see if we can deal with the leftover feelings before we talk about how the decision was made. Does that sound okay? [*The group nods in agreement*]. Mathew, you said you wanted to add something?

Mathew: Yes, thanks, Paul. I just want everyone to know that Marie and I understand and accept that Nicole had to leave camp. She brought drugs to camp, which is a clear violation of our policies. And she was also in violation of her probation, and that had to be reported. It was just hard that we were not told the facts right at the beginning.

[*Turning to Celeste*]: You let us think she was having a nervous breakdown, and naturally, we were upset that anyone would send her away from camp if that was the problem.

Marie: And while you told us one story, everyone else knew the real story. How do you think that made me feel when I found out the young adults knew Nicole brought drugs to camp and here I am, her grandmother, and I don't know a single thing about it!

Celeste [*speaking through tears*]: I know I should have told you right away. I was so ashamed and worried that you would think all of this was my fault 'cause of Stan. I mean, I know how upset you are about the divorce, and then this happens the first time you finally came back to camp. I was just so ashamed.

Nelson: Mathew and Marie, I can imagine how hard it must have been for you during the time you didn't know what was going on. I think we were all remiss in just assuming Celeste would be able to tell you about it.

[*Turning to Celeste*]: I remember how upset and ashamed you were, Celeste, and I wish we had picked up on that better, or that you had had the trust to ask us to help you.

Celeste [*still in tears*]: I know I could have asked. [*Looking at Maura*]: It's not like Maura and Eliana didn't offer. I just did not want to face it. Here I was, this mother who did all these things before that everyone gossiped about, and now it's my kid who has to leave camp because she's a druggie. You have no idea how awful that was. . . .

Marie [*leaning toward Celeste*]: Celeste, it is not your fault that Nicole decided to take drugs again. I personally think you did the right thing letting the Committee know that she had violated her probation. Without those limits, I think she would have just gone on fooling everyone, and now she is getting the help she needs. Yes, I'm upset, but it's because I didn't know what was going on and when I finally did get the information, I found out that just about everyone else in camp already knew. And that was just hard to take. I just cannot understand how you could be so dishonest with us!

Mathew: I also agree that it was important that you told the Executives about Nicole violating her probation. I really do accept that she had to leave camp. I just can't accept that you had to lie to us about it. I mean, we aren't that judgmental, are we?

Celeste is in tears and unable to respond.

Maura: You know, Mathew and Marie, I don't think this is just about Nicole and camp and Stan and all that.

[*Turning and taking Celeste's hand*]: Celeste, you have done a lot of work at camp over the years, and it feels to me that what is happening now is as much about your family-of-origin issues as about what happened at camp this year. . . . Do you think?

Celeste: You mean the little kid who is always causing trouble and always being rejected? [*Laughing with some bitterness*]:

Yeah, you might say those issues have come up a lot lately. I knew the minute I told Mathew and Marie that Nicole left because she was too upset that I had done it again. I was not being honest with them, and that would get them upset and mad. The funny thing is that was the one thing I was trying to avoid. Talk about being self-defeating! But I just felt that they would be so angry . . . first the divorce and now this.

Mike: Celeste, whatever we felt about the divorce and you marrying Stan is done and over with. We would not have decided to come back to camp if we had not been able to put that behind us. Sure, we were disappointed at first. It's always hard to see marriages end and even harder when it involves your children. But we know you are happy. Yes, we think things have been hard for Nicole, but we also hope that maybe now that she is older, she can learn how to handle her life a little better. Believe me, any upset we had at camp was not because we were mad about you getting together with Stan.

Paul: Celeste, does that make things clearer for you?

Celeste: I guess so. [*Looking around the group*]: I just want to apologize to everyone for making things such a mess at camp.

Maura: You know, I don't think things were that much of a mess. It was hard that people had information they couldn't discuss as a community, but I think people understood that your family needed to work things out before we could do anything as a community.

Paul: Okay, are we ready to move on to the second part of this discussion—how the decision to tell Nicole she had to leave was made? [*The group agrees*]. Just so everyone has the same information, I want to start by reviewing the information we had when we made the decision.

This is the third time Nicole brought marijuana to camp. The first two times, the young adult group handled the issue. On both those occasions, Celeste and Stan were told what happened and they agreed they would help Nicole get treatment. Nita checked with Nicole and her parents during each year after she used at camp. Nicole was in treatment, and Nita felt the issue had been handled.

When we got this report, both Nita and Lincoln recommended that the consequence for her actions had to be implemented, and the Executive Committee agreed. I also think it is fair to say that Nicole violating her probation made the issue feel more urgent. [*Looking to the other members of the Executive Committee*]: Does anyone else want to add anything else?

Maura: Well, I think the timing of how things went is also important. We got the information from Celeste at our first morning meeting [of the Executive Committee and therapists], on Sunday before Temperature Reading. So we met with Nicole, who did not deny that she had been using marijuana. We explained why she needed to leave and, although she was pretty upset, she did agree to leave. Then we talked about how to let the community know and decided Eliana and Paul would make the announcement at Temperature Reading while Lincoln and Nita met with Nicole and Celeste to talk about who would talk with Stan and Mathew and Marie.

James [*interrupting*]: I think that's where the process broke down. I don't understand why you didn't meet with the full Committee before telling Nicole to leave. Then at least there would have been more community input, and if it seemed right, we could have decided to take the issue to the whole community.

Several people begin to talk at once. Paul asks people to raise their hands to speak, and he turns to Nelson first.

Nelson: It really wasn't a decision I would have taken to the community. It involved things that had been confidential to the young adults group, and there were family members who needed to be told what happen. It was also important that the consequence happen right away.

Maura: I feel okay about how we handled the issue with Nicole, but I feel less sure about how we handled the issue with the community. I do think the problem we had was not meeting right away with the Committee so that you had the information and understood our decision-making process. I believe we had good intentions . . . we wanted to give Celeste time to talk with Mathew and Marie before we gave the information to more people. What we didn't understand was how difficult that would be for Celeste. But we didn't follow up on the family, and it was Wednesday when Mathew and Marie talked with Eliana and she realized they did not have all of the information.

Marie: And of course, by then we were pretty upset. To be honest, I did not want to have any more discussion after we finally found out what was going on. I'm glad it was not a subject for the whole community, and I think even a Committee meeting would have been awfully hard to take.

Sissy: Well, I understand how you feel. It was difficult for me when I realized you didn't have the full story about what had happened with Nicole. I wanted to tell you myself, but I knew that was not my place.

Serena: Well, I for one didn't have all this information. I felt like the situation was handled, and I was really okay with that. I think it helped that people talked about how they were feeling at the first work session. I figured the Execs would handle it during camp, and we would talk about it here. Personally, I don't think everyone has to know everything all the time. I know we are supposed to process things that affect the community, but a lot of time I think people just want to get information so they can be in on the gossip.

James: I totally disagree. This is a camp based on Satir philosophy and methods, and Virginia believed that there is nothing that can't be handled when people have the skills and support that they need. Not telling the community is like keeping a secret in the family.

Maura: Some of that is true, James, but I'm not sure that always taking individual issues to the entire camp is the best way to handle things, particularly when there are problems families may not be ready to talk about. We all know that in the past, some people have been badly hurt and even left our community when we have taken things to the whole group and they were not handled well. I think the decision we made was right for Nicole and her family. I don't believe taking that kind of issue to the whole community was necessary for them or for the community.

Denise: I also think we have to acknowledge the therapists' role in this decision. As I understand it, the therapists were the first to recommend that Nicole be told to leave, is that right?

Sondra: That's right. Both Lincoln and Nita felt that we had to hold to the agreements that were made the last time Nicole relapsed at camp. And then Eliana felt strongly that the legal issue had to be resolved.

Denise: We have to respect the therapists' decision about how they want to work with people in camp. Nicole is someone who has been getting therapeutic help for several years here at camp. As far as I can tell, this was a therapeutic decision as much as it was a decision related to camp policy.

James: So does that mean we have no say, when the therapists decide, it's "therapeutically necessary"?

Denise: Are you asking do I think we have to defer to them when there is a therapeutic issue? Absolutely. That's why we hire them.

Sissy: But what if the Executive Committee did not want to tell Nicole to leave?

Sondra: I think that could have happened under a different set of circumstances and they would have processed the issue with the therapists until they reached a consensus. In this case, there was consensus about the therapeutic issue as well as the needs of camp. The Executive Committee felt Nicole's behavior put the camp at risk, and she had to leave for that reason as well as for violating her treatment agreement.

James: But that decision was huge for the community, and only a very small group of people got to make it.

Paul: I agree, and that's why I would like us to look at how we could have kept the Committee informed during this process so that the group as a whole can be involved when something this significant happens.

Alta: Well, I'm okay with the Executives and facilitators handling the information in private and making that decision because it had to be made so quickly. I think if there had been time for more process, then the whole Committee being involved might have made sense. But in this case, I also think it would have helped if the Executives had met with the Committee early in the week, like Tuesday or Wednesday, and gave the Committee some sense of what was going on. The information had already been shared with the young adult group, and we as a Committee could have helped camp feel more comfortable if we had had the information.

I'm not suggesting that we needed a full discussion at Temperature Reading, but we could have assured people who spoke to us individually that we knew what was going on and that we agreed with the decision. In reality, we were asking the camp to trust us to handle an issue that was private to one family. And that is what we usually do, but this time the Committee didn't have any information on which to ask for that trust.

Serena: I think I get what you mean, Alta. I know I heard bits and pieces of the story, but I would have been clearer and able to say to people, "Look, it's okay, the Execs did what they had to do" if I knew what had happened. I don't mean before the decision was made. Just that we had talked it through and understood why the decision had been made. For instance, I didn't know that Nicole had been told that if she smoked dope again, she would be asked to leave. That makes a big difference to how I see the situation.

Paul: What I hear is that big decisions like this need to be shared and understood by the entire Committee, not just the Execs. Unfortunately, I think we got caught up in the family struggle and lost sight of the impact on the community. I understand what you mean, Alta, about how you and others can help the whole camp feel better when you know what is going on. And when the Committee takes on that role, then we don't always have to process everything in the big group.

Charles: Well, I guess I agree. I'm sure even Virginia knew about stuff that was going on and just handled it rather than bringing every single problem to the big group.

Athena: I agree, Charles. I think it is important to see how much progress we have made as a community since Virginia left. Today we processed some old stuff that has been hard for a lot of us. It means a lot to me, Mathew and

Marie, that you have come back to camp and that you were able to support Celeste today. I think you three talking together brings healing to all of us who have felt divided by what has happened to your family. I also think that we have made progress as a community because we are thinking about how we deal with therapeutic issues and community issues.

Don't forget that Family Camp was one big experiment to Virginia. She wanted to see what would happen when she applied her theories and methods about families at a community level. We need to remember even Virginia didn't really know what would work or not work. It was all trial and error, and we are continuing her experiment. However, we have had more time to practice and learn from what we do.

I think this past camp was an example of the Committee and the Execs doing just what they should do. The therapists helped a family support and care for a member who has a substance abuse problem. At the same time, the Execs made a decision to protect the community. Not all of that required the involvement of the whole community. This began as a family issue and when it affected camp, the body responsible for protecting camp took the appropriate action. Yes, we probably need to do a better job at keeping the whole Committee informed, but overall, I think Virginia would have both agreed with the decision and also been pleased at the process and how the family as well as the community was both supported and protected.

After much time and effort, the Committee resolved most of the concerns that were created by Nicole's behavior and its aftermath. This experience deepened the Committee's understanding of the delicate balance required to maintain a family's confidentiality and the community's need to deal with issues that affect the community as a whole. As an *sfc* camper and former board member reflected,

> Working with therapeutic issues at the community level has been an evolving process at camp. Developing and supporting a community requires a systems approach that can recognize patterns and address issues that provide an opportunity for community growth. We've become pretty good at identifying and dealing with issues that

threaten the community, and I think we are getting better at trying to deal with those issues before they get to the level of a threat. One of the things that gets in the way of sfc growing as a community is a lot of the old baggage people are carrying around. It is difficult to process and reach consensus in a community when people are attaching old angers and hurts from the past to the issue of today. What I feel positive about is that sfc is a conscious community, and with effective leadership and skilled facilitators, we can and do make anything work.

Another camper and current board member said:

Therapeutic issues at camp are so complicated. Every time an individual deals with issues, the community is affected in some way. It is also important for us to know that camp itself has its dark side, just as most individuals do. What makes us succeed as a community is that we look at our dark side and shine a light on it. We also work very hard to deal with our dark side. We keep learning, and each time we go through a struggle on a community level, we get stronger as individuals and as a community.

Confronting Each Other and Surviving as a Community

Examining the dark side of camp often involves the community being willing not only to discuss but also confront the darkness in individuals and in the group as a whole. In contrast to the Virginia-led camp, when issues that Virginia saw as important to the community were identified and addressed by the community at large, the post-Virginia Family Camp has found addressing issues at a community level one of the most challenging parts of the camp experience. The confrontation with Mick, along with other somewhat less dramatic events, have made the community wary of facing issues that involve intense conflict, particularly in unstructured settings. During the period of stagnation described at the beginning of this chapter, people made a deliberate effort to maintain stability at camp. This stifled not only creativity but also discontent. Issues surfaced through individual or family work or at a special-interest group. Few if any issues arose spontaneously, and if they did, they were quickly taken into a more controlled setting. When the teen group identified under-age drinking, a planned response was created by organizing a work session about communication among the teens and their parents. When the drinking at camp continued and became even more complicated by adult use of illegal substances at camp, the issue again went to a work session followed by discussion at the November Committee meeting. At no time did the community at large address these contentious issues, despite the fact that some teenagers in camp passed out from excessive drinking, and despite some Committee members being among the adults using drugs.

In contrast, the following event regarding whether to allow filming at camp began at Temperature Reading and involved the full community throughout the decision-making process. This is a recreation of an actual event at the 2004 camp. We have changed names to maintain confidentiality.

To Film or Not to Film

Three weeks before the 2004 Family Camp, one of the four facilitators, Eliana, called the Committee vice president, Connie, to discuss a proposal for filming at camp.

Eliana: Connie, I have such great news.

Connie: What's up?

Eliana: Well, Rob Schmidt contacted me just today. Do you know Rob?

Connie: No, should I?

Eliana: Well, maybe not . . . he is just this wonderful dear man who knew Virginia for years and years and also attended camp in the early days. Anyway, he is working with a film company that is producing a film about Virginia and her work. Isn't that wonderful?

Connie: Definitely! I think it's great that Virginia's work will get some recognition. So, is this going to involve camp in some way?

Eliana: That's the best part of the news! Rob and I talked, and we agreed that we should include something about Family Camp in the film. And with camp happening in the next few weeks, I thought we could invite him to come to camp and film what we do. What do you think?

Connie: Well, personally, I think it would be important that camp get included in a film about Virginia's work, but you know I can't make that decision, Eliana, and neither can you. We need to talk to the Committee, and we also need to discuss it with the whole camp before we just have him arrive. Remember how concerned everyone gets even when old campers come back to visit without any announcement?

Eliana: Yes, but I'm sure there won't be any problem with Rob. After all, he used to be a camper.

Connie: I'll tell you what I can do. I'll e-mail the Committee and tell them about the film and your idea about including sfc as well as having Rob film at camp, and let's see what kind of reaction we get.

The Committee's initial reaction was mixed. Most members were interested in exploring the idea, but some felt concern about the timing. Many members thought the full camp would not have time to discuss the idea, reach a decision, and then (assuming the community agrees) arrange the filming. Some Committee members suggested that the community discuss the proposal at the 2004 camp and, if they agreed, do the filming at the 2005 camp. That option was ruled out quickly because the entire film, including the sfc portion, had to be finished by the end of the 2004 calendar year.

Another problem was that Eliana had tentatively scheduled the filming for Wednesday, which meant the community needed to decide by Tuesday. Most Committee members knew that any idea that affected how camp operates could require lots of processing before the community would be ready to make a decision.

The first Temperature Reading of the 2004 camp occurred on Sunday morning. During the time set aside for "New Information," Eliana enthusiastically announced that there would be film made about Virginia's life and that the filmmaker had invited sfc to participate in that film. The first campers to respond to the announcement expressed pride that Family Camp had received the invitation and enthusiastically endorsed the camp's participation. As generally happens at Temperature Reading, the more people stood up and spoke in favor of participating in the film, the more it appeared that the group was reaching a consensus. The camp president and leader of Sunday's Temperature Reading, attempted to sum up:

Carl: Well, it looks like many people are in favor of doing the film. Can we get a few volunteers to work with Eliana on ideas for what we want to have filmed? Then they can bring their recommendations back here tomorrow and we can make a final decision on how to do this.

At that moment, the quiet murmur that has been underlying the more overt positive comments becomes a chorus of "Wait a minute" and "Not so fast."

Maura: I know we've been discussing this proposal for a long time, and many of you want to get on with camp, but I really don't support filming at camp. I also know lots of you think this is a wonderful idea, so it's hard for me to speak against something a lot of people want to do. But I need to express my concerns.

I am not comfortable with someone coming into camp and filming what happens here. Allowing that will have a negative effect on what I want to happen at camp, for me. This is a week where I want to be totally free to be me. I want to be able to express what I want the way I want. To do that, I have to know that there is safety here. When I know there is safety, then I have the freedom to be me. But when we talk about having someone come in and filming camp, my sense of safety disappears. I'm not sure I know why I feel that way, I just do.

Cynthia: Thank you, Maura, for standing up and saying what a lot of us are feeling. I feel like a train is about to run me over. I'm glad that Virginia's work will be recognized, but I do not understand why this one week we have at camp has to be affected——

Stan [*interrupting in a patronizing tone*]: Because camp was a big part of Virginia's work, and if a film is being made about that work, then we should be included. In case you don't know, camp is one part of Virginia's work that even some of her closest colleagues know almost nothing about. This film will give us the opportunity to not only tell about her work but also actually show it!

Cynthia: Stan, you may feel that way, but I do not. I don't want to be shown.

Stan: Then don't participate.

Cynthia: So what do I do, go hide while the filming goes on?

Stan: You don't have to hide. You can just go be in a part of camp that isn't being filmed!

Cynthia [*sarcastically*]: Well isn't that just a great idea. I will just go off and be ostracized from the group. [*She turns to the group as a whole and speaks with more emotion*]: I struggle with feeling excluded all year, and camp is the one place and the one time of year when I can count on being included. I come here because I know this is where I will be valued and loved for who I am. Now I feel like you want to take that away from me!

Anita: I just find this whole discussion upsetting. Cynthia just wants to come to camp and have the experience she waits all year for, and then you [*to Stan*] tell her, "Just don't participate." Can't you see how excluding that is? Why would we deliberately do something at camp that sets up divisions among us when what we say we want is to build a community that is very inclusive?

Maura: But I can see that if we *don't* do the filming, then we are preventing some of the community from participating in something that has great meaning for them, and that isn't what we want in our community, either.

Alisa: Is coming to camp and filming the only way that sfc can participate in Virginia's film? Isn't there some way that people who want to could be interviewed without the filming being intrusive to others who do not want to participate? On the other hand, what about using still pictures of things here at camp along with interviews? I just don't think filming is the only option we have.

Eliana: We could do that, but to understand sfc, you have to actually see camp and what goes on here. Like when the kids are swinging on the rope over there, and how people take time to talk or read or play and, of course, how we process things at Temperature Reading. It would be so much richer to see camp operate than just talk about it or show photographs. But that is another way we could do it.

Maura: I guess I just have trouble understanding how people would not be uncomfortable having some stranger—okay, I know Rob knows camp, but he is still a stranger to most of us. I just don't understand how it can be such a dilemma for me and not a problem for others.

Nita: What I hear you saying, Maura—and others as well—is that camp has a sacred place in your heart that is important because it makes you safe to be you. Moreover, that safety is dependent upon camp being open and yet at the same time protected. And if there is someone in camp who comes as an observer to take pictures, even if you are not in those pictures, some of that safety is removed.

Maura: Yes, that's it. And I get that part, but how is it that others are not as affected by the outsider coming in as I am?

Alisa: I feel that need for safety, too. The safety allows us to be so open with each other and ourselves. However, I feel it mostly at sessions. I feel less disrupted by people visiting or participating with us in our general living activities.

Sean: I come to camp to relax and be with people I like and enjoy. I guess for me, the safety issue is a given. People who come to camp commit themselves to our values and our process, and I just assume camp is safe. But I know I also don't take a lot of risks here, which makes this less of a big deal for me.

Ben: I guess I'm in a different place because I know Rob Schmidt. I was here when he was a camper. He is a quiet, unassuming guy who is really committed to Virginia and maintaining her legacy. He knows what camp is and I see him like me, just another guy taking pictures.

Cynthia: Well, I don't know him, and the idea of another guy "just taking pictures" makes me uncomfortable. What if we work out the most careful plan and he still films someone who does not want to be in the film? Then what? Will we get to edit the film?

Eliana: We could certainly ask for that, and I'm sure he will agree.

Alisa: I have a different problem with this whole thing. I'm concerned about the process. I think, given time, camp could find a compromise that would work for everyone. But this is a really complicated issue for us. We are talking about serious stuff: about safety, inclusion, and exclusion. And I feel we don't have the time we need to process all of this in the time frame that was given us.

Eliana: I wish that I had heard about this earlier, but you know, Rob just called me in May, and at that point he hadn't even thought about including camp. It was my suggestion that he use the time he was going to spend interviewing me to add something about camp.

Stan: See, no one even thought about including camp. So no wonder we don't have much time. But it just makes it all the more important that we do this so people know about sfc and how important it was to Virginia.

Nita: What I hear are different needs and desires that appear to conflict. I wonder if we can first get clear about the issues. Then maybe we can begin to process those issues and see where there is or is not consensus. Here's what I think I have heard so far.

- Having a film made at camp would not interfere with some people's experience of camp.
- For others, camp is a sacred place that should be shared only with those who are present and participating in the experience. For these people, having a film made during camp would interfere with what they need and want from camp.
- We all value Virginia's work and want to see it honored by a film and want to see sfc included in that film.
- We differ on how to include sfc in the film itself.
- Those who support filming at camp want to show how camp operates so that people can see how Virginia's work continues to this day.
- People who oppose filming at camp want to see sfc included in a film but want to have that happen in a way that does not involve filming during camp.
- People are concerned about being heard and having their views understood and respected during this process.

Although there is some discussion after Nita's summation, most people are getting frustrated by the discussion and want to move on into camp activities.

Nelson: I think we need to move on and start camp, but I also know that this is an issue that will consume us if we don't take care of it now. I am willing to work with a smaller group to talk about the things that Nita identified and see if we can bring back some suggestions to the whole group tomorrow.

Eliana: That sounds good to me. How about people who want to work on this issue meet with me right after Temperature Reading and we can set a time this afternoon to process this more and see if we can bring a possible consensus to the larger group?

A small group of people representing different viewpoints volunteered. That group met after lunch. Although the group represented a variety of viewpoints about how to achieve the goal, the majority began from the position of wanting to have the camp included in the film. This working group took the time it needed to have all of the participants explain their reasons for supporting or opposing filming at camp. The process clarified the various ways that people experience camp. It also helped clarify how intensely the filming made some campers feel both vulnerable and unsafe.

As those wanting to film at camp became aware of others' feelings of vulnerability, they stepped back from the view that those opposed to filming were trying to prevent camp's involvement in the film. They became less rigid and more willing to discuss ways to achieve a compromise. Although a few on the other side did not move from their total opposition to the filming, most were more willing to negotiate a compromise.

At Monday's Temperature Reading, the working group returned to the whole community with several ideas for a compromise. Several members of the small group summarized the process that occurred during their first meeting. Those supporting the filming discussed its importance for the camp but acknowledged that there are ways to participate in the film while lessening the impact on camp. Those opposed to the filming articulated their concerns with more clarity and presented suggestions for how filming might be least disruptive to their camp experience.

Following this discussion, the ever-pragmatic Sean suggested that the community choose among the following options:

1. Camp members would be interviewed on camera, but still pictures and other material about camp would be provided to the filmmaker; and no filming would happen during or at camp.
2. Filming would occur that week but at a site outside of camp.

3. Filming would occur at camp on Wednesday in a restricted setting.
4. Filming would occur at camp on Wednesday and the film-maker would have open access to all parts of camp.

He then suggested a straw vote to find out where people stood at that moment. To facilitate voting, someone drew a line in the dirt in front of the amphitheater and put cross-hatches on the line to represent the four options. To vote, campers stood at the marked places. On the first vote, the majority stood at spots 2, 3, or 4. Cynthia stood alone on spot 1.

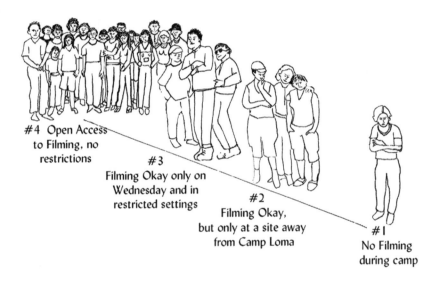

#4 Open Access to Filming, no restrictions

#3 Filming Okay only on Wednesday and in restricted settings

#2 Filming Okay, but only at a site away from Camp Loma

#1 No Filming during camp

When Anita realized Cynthia was standing alone and in tears, she quickly joined her. Other family members and friends then joined them. As people changed their positions on the line, it became apparent that the camp was splitting into factions. The straw vote demonstrated that as long as even one member stood on option 1, the camp could not reach a consensus.

Heated discussion began regarding how camp makes decisions. At this point, the community was stymied regarding its position on whether decisions are by majority rule or total consensus. The discussion grew more and more fractious.

Nita: I want the camp to recognize that we are discussing more than just who supports and who opposes filming at camp or how the camp makes decisions. I hear people speaking about feelings of trust and questioning whether they can be safe at camp. When these concerns are raised, we need to slow down and listen very carefully, even if only one voice out of the entire community is speaking about these issues.

Eliana: When I first heard about the film, I was excited, even passionate, about the opportunity to show the world SFC. But as I have participated in this process, both here at Temperature Reading and in the small group meetings, I realize that my passion about sharing Virginia's work has gotten in the way of my hearing all your voices and understanding how different camp is for each of you.

Nita is right. When just one person at camp talks of losing trust and not having safety at camp, we must all listen. How can we say we are living Virginia's principles if we do not respect each voice and every need here at camp?

I know if feels unfair to the majority that one person can stop what so many other people want to have happen at camp. But we know that there are many ways that SFC can be included in the film. What I now understand is there is no way to have filming at camp and assure that every single person feels safe and included in camp.

Therefore, because I am the person who was invited to participate in the film and brought this idea to camp, I am going to ask you to support me in making the decision. As long as there is even one person who is uncomfortable with filming during camp, we will not film at camp. That does not mean SFC will not be in the film. I want to continue to figure out a way to do that. But for now, I want to call Rob and tell him not to come Wednesday and also tell him that we will get back to him about ways that we agree camp can be included in the film.

By this time, most of the community was seriously divided about the issue and frustrated with the process. It was clear that they could not reach a 100-percent consensus about filming by the deadline, the next day, without spending most of Monday on this issue. Since the community lacked enough energy to continue the process, people accepted Eliana's request/decision. Even after that, some parts of the community struggled about the choice. Throughout the week, people spent time discussing different parts of the issue, and the community reached a deeper understanding about what had happened. At the final work session, the processing that had occurred all week was reflected in Vince's closing comments:

> Most of you know that I have been struggling all week about the decision we made about the film. You also know that I initially supported the filming because it made sense to me and it was very important to my wife. When we took the straw vote, it became a personal issue, because I saw the will of the majority being thwarted by a very small number of people. When we originally voted, only one person opposed the filming. All the other campers were willing to let it happen. Yet it did not happen.
>
> So, most of the week, I've been pissed because it seems like camp has rejected the principle of majority rule. That principle is very important to me. I try to live by democratic principles in all my life, and especially at camp.
>
> Then I sat down with Maura, and I think I finally got it. There is another equally important principle in our community: that we as a community both support and care for every member, whether we agree with them or not. And it is that principle which makes us truly unique. For some people, this issue is much more than whether there should be filming at camp. For them, it is about safety and being heard. And if an issue leaves even one member of camp unheard or unsafe, then our entire community cannot be safe. When we are discussing that kind of issue, there can be no majority rule. Either everyone feels safe or no one is safe. Once I understood that, I understood that we made the right decision, and I am not only resolved about the decision, I also feel good about the process we used to get to resolution.

In the end, the community did find a solution that allowed the filming to happen. Camp ended on Saturday, and those who wanted and were able to participate in the filming were invited to stay at camp after the closing session. Filming occurred at camp in areas that were still set up but no longer officially part of camp. As past president, Maura participated in the filming and felt resolved about the outcome. Cynthia and Anita did not.

The decision about filming forced the community to resolve the conflict between the needs of a few individuals for strong boundaries at camp with the majority's desire to have filming occur during camp.

In the process, this helped the entire community understand the importance of boundaries and safety at camp. The community also learned more about how it makes decisions when one individual's needs seem pitted against the will of the majority. Most important, the community addressed a contentious and difficult issue in an open and often uncontrolled environment. During this week, various people expressed very strong feelings and were both angry and hurt. Not everyone was satisfied or felt comfortable with the outcome, but for the first time in many years the community both identified and dealt with an issue as a community rather than as groups of individuals.

Inclusion, Exclusion, and an Intentional Community Issue

One of the most vexing issues for SFC, as it is for most intentional communities, continues to be members' feelings of inclusion and exclusion. The mission statement says that SFC offers a place where "every individual from infant to elder is known, appreciated, and respected for his or her unique contributions and inherent goodness." Yet, every year, the camp struggles to implement this principle. Often, the feelings of exclusion are self-generated, as demonstrated in this story about Liz, who has attended camp for over ten years. Letisha is the therapist facilitating a meeting of the women's group. The story is a recreation of actual events, and the names are fictitious.

A Cafeteria Moment

Letisha [*therapist*]: Liz had something that bubbled up for her today and would like time to talk about. Shall we begin there? [*The group agrees*].

Liz: I'm just feeling so disconnected and not a part of this group anymore. The last couple of years, I tell myself I'm just too busy to attend, but this year I realized it's not that I'm busy, it's really I just don't think I have a place here. It is so difficult for me to see where I fit anymore. Here I am turning 64, my kids are grown and on their own, and when I think about being part of this group, I just feel like I'm 16 and back in high school.

[*Turning to the young woman next to her*]: You know, Charlene, I just don't know how to relate to you, [*looking at the group's other women in their 20s*]: or any of you. I feel like

I walk into the bathroom and if you are in there, particularly if you are standing around in a group, I just want to go out the door. Sometimes I find myself just staying in the stall, hoping you will leave so I won't have to come out and . . . I guess, be ignored or feel stupid or not know what to say.

[*The young women in the group look both startled and slightly embarrassed*].

I'm not saying you do anything wrong or that you do anything at all. I know my reaction is about me and what I'm feeling. It's like, here are all these popular, gorgeous girls and here am I, the total dork. And, god, I'm over 60, not 16!!!

Several of the older women laugh and agree.

Sherry: Liz, I have had exactly the same feeling. Yesterday in the bathroom, I came out of the stall talking about how I was worried the toilet would overflow, and there were three of the teenagers standing there looking at me like I was this creature from Mars. Finally, Megan asked me if I was okay, and I just kind of laughed and said, "Oh, yeah" and rushed away. I felt like such an idiot!

The group held further discussion about times people felt uncomfortable in camp. Several younger women shared their confusion about how to relate with older campers whom they do not know well. Letisha then joined in.

Letisha: What I hear people talking about is not being sure if they have a place in camp. First, Liz talked about feeling detached from the women in camp. Then others talked about the challenges of relating to each other across the age groups. What I hear beneath these issues is a more fundamental question about belonging: do we really belong here? Is there room for me? Can I be part of this group?

Lee Ann: You know, for me, it happens when I go to meals. Most of the time, I go with Manny and we sit together but, like, yesterday he was doing his job and there I was, I had my plate and I turned around and all of sudden, I had this, like, "Cafeteria Moment." You know, when you were in high school and you had to decide where you were going to sit in the cafeteria? [*Loud laughter follows as the women become aware of how this "Cafeteria Moment" captures their universal fear and longing to belong*].

People join intentional communities to be part of a group that promises inclusion. Often, people hide their feelings of self-generated exclusion, as Liz did, under the guise of being busy. Or, as Letisha pointed out, they put their feelings on top of other feelings. However, when the issue "bubbles up" as it did for Liz, an intentional community such as sfc can provide the forum and the support to help members address the issue even if they are not aware of what is causing the feeling. As Liz recounted:

> That year at women's group, I got back in touch with how I was feeling disconnected at camp. I really thought I had worked out my fear of being rejected and being an outsider. It used to be that every year I came to camp, I was full of dread about being in a group of over a hundred people! Then I got involved with the Committee and volunteered for lots of jobs at camp, and I felt part of things. I told myself that I was too busy to go to women's group any more. Finally, I admitted it was more than that. I decided to go to the women's group that day to talk about something very different. I had no idea that I no longer felt part of the group because of my age until I started talking about how hard it is for me to relate to the younger women. And then to hear that Sherry and other women felt the same way made me feel less like an outsider. Then Letisha helped us see that we all were talking about that old fear of "do I really belong?" That's why Lee Ann's "Cafeteria Moment" just resonated so strongly with all of us. We all knew what we were talking about, and suddenly the walls came down. That day in that group, I totally got in touch with the magic of a camp!

Camp Governance

The sfc community also continues to struggle with issues related to camp governance, particularly its leadership. For the past decade, with few exceptions, the same people have served on the Committee. This has had both advantages and disadvantages for the community as a whole. The fact that some people are willing to volunteer many hours of their time, physical labor and, on occasion, money, is a major reason why sfc has both survived and thrived. The individuals responsible for running camp have longevity both as campers and members of the governing body, which has provided stability in times of crises. This consistent group of volunteers has also developed shared wisdom and an ability to work together effectively.

On the other hand, the entrenchment of the Committee members, particularly the officers, has led to struggles within sfc. Although people are encouraged to serve on the Committee, in reality, most of the officers' roles have remained within a select group and not available to new people. In 2003, several members of the community raised the issue of term limits for the officers' positions.

This suggestion resulted in acrimonious and painful discussions at Committee meetings that year. Feelings became so heated that the president requested the assistance of an organizational consultant (and sfc camper) to help Committee members process the issue. Committee members recognized that serving on the Committee and as an officer came with lots of work and little reward. At the same time, they also acknowledged that they continue being part of the Committee because of the pleasure of the support they get from being part of the group and having more contact with camp throughout the year. Through this discussion, the Committee recognized that long-term membership on the Executive Committee had created issues of inclusion and exclusion for some campers. They also saw that the struggle around term limits pointed to ongoing issues that the Committee needed to address.

The Committee agreed that more than one of its members need to have both the knowledge about and experience with executive functions. Although the Committee did not adopt term limits, it did agree to train new people about the governance of camp, including finances, registration, and record keeping. Not all of the anger and hurt generated by this discussion was resolved, however, and at least one member of the Executive Committee chose to resign and to leave camp.

Equally important, the year-long discussion about term limits also led the Committee to increase the involvement of more campers in camp governance. Recognizing that most campers participate in only the week-long camp, several Committee members looked at how to change operations at camp to enhance people's involvement. Traditionally, the Committee had been responsible for both opening and closing camp. These two tasks involve a great deal of work by a small group of people, particularly at the week's end, when most people are tired and facing long drives home. Following the term-limits discussion, two Committee members drew up a list of tasks that all camp members could complete to close camp. In a major shift of responsibility and work, the Committee decided to share the closing of camp with the whole community.

In some ways, this is a small and logical shift in how the work is done. In other ways, it is a significant recognition that during camp, the entire community can and should be more responsible for it.

Community Implications

The Satir Family Camp community as it exists today is moving from the stage of Status Quo into Ennui. During the past few years, the community has been willing to look at its actions and be responsible for identifying, naming, and changing behaviors. As it has matured, the community's ability to consider individual and collective higher-level needs has increased. The community long ago moved from a focus on survival—setting up shelter, food, and water stations from its time at Pico Blanco—and reached a level of performance that equitably supports the needs of most members. In this state, more energy is available to focus on individual growth and community issues around relationships.

Some of the behaviors the community has examined are: exclusion and inclusion within the camp, inconsistent policies, and favored and nonfavored members. Each time people name and confront one of these behaviors or issues, the community has strengthened its commitment to its fundamental principles. Much of the focus in the past few years has been on creating a process that supports open debate and shared decision making.

To combat the boredom and stagnation common to this stage of development, SFC has worked hard to modify its structure. Previously mentioned examples are reconstituting the Pulse Committee and creating exercises such as the mixed-group lunch discussion held at the 2005 camp. These aimed to minimize the growing separation among the camp's subgroups. In earlier developmental stages, the community's energy and effort would never have focused on relieving boredom and stagnation, because when survival is at stake, there is little room for ennui. For instance, at Pico Blanco, people devoted energy to meeting their survival needs in an isolated place without with any modern conveniences. Indeed, that site needed work just for people to make it through the week on a very simple level. Campers divided their energy between survival and growth.

Camp Loma, by contrast, meets campers' needs with the modern conveniences of an existing, year-round site with many luxurious recreational amenities such as ping pong, swimming, and volleyball. The very nature of the camp location and facility freed up energy to focus on things other than mere survival.

Departing from the large-group identity and work sessions and moving toward special-interest groups such as women's group and men's group is also consistent with the developmental stage of Ennui. With less energy focused on survival, community members can join with others with whom they have much in common: age, family status, interests, and so on. In earlier stages of development, the common interests are survival and then fundamental functions. In later stages, such as Synergy and finally Ennui, the community's structure is not only defined but operating successfully to meet the primary and more advanced needs of its members.

By utilizing Satir principles and methods, camp has, to date, avoided being thrown back into Rebellion as is common when a community becomes too stagnant. The plan for the future will have to consider how to avoid and/or negotiate Rebellion in the coming years as the need for change reemerges. What remains consistent is Virginia's belief that growth is always possible and light should be shined into even the darkest corners. This principle remains as her legacy in SFC.

7

The Struggle with Ennui

As SFC moved from the stage of Synergy to Ennui, it increased its ability to integrate new ideas and also to cope with larger changes that inevitably face all communities. One of these is mortality. Over its many years of existence, a few SFC campers have died from illness and accidents. Many campers who left SFC when Virginia left have died in old age, but not until 2005 did campers who had been part of the community since its beginnings have to leave because of age. Soon after, they died. The following stories honor two such campers; only their names differ.

SFC **Angels**

Calvin and his wife Marnie joined SFC during the early Pico Blanco years. Marnie found the therapeutic program fascinating and soaked up Virginia's teachings and ideas for herself as well as for her professional work. Calvin was active in the more practical side of camp. At Pico Blanco, he was one of Harry's primary assistants. When SFC moved to Camp Loma, Calvin took over Harry's role as the camp caretaker. He did necessary chores and solved the numerous logistical problems that inevitably occur during camp. When something did not work or a problem needed solving, the cry went out, "Where's Calvin?" With few exceptions, Calvin soon fixed it.

Each year when members of the Committee arrived a day early to set up Camp Loma, Calvin's Subaru would already be near the entrance. He was the first to arrive and the last to leave, making sure that the camp was open and the Committee had everything necessary to start preparations. In the year between camps, Calvin also served as the liaison between the owners of Camp Loma and the Committee. This entailed going to the camp grounds to deal with the effects of winter storms on the land and the buildings. As one Committee member recalled:

> It seemed to me that Calvin single-handedly managed the physical part of camp. I remember him, at age 70, climbing up on the roof of the latrines to fix a leak or hiking up into the hills to unblock the stream that fed the pool.

A camper said:

> Calvin was such a quiet presence at camp. He didn't always speak out, but you always knew he was involved with what was going on. He would attend all the work sessions, sitting in the front row next to Marnie. When I did work, I could always look down and there he would be, smiling up at me, just radiating care and support.

Another camper related:

> My enduring memory of Calvin was his role as "Camp Dad." For so many years, when the person working was asked to pick out someone to be their dad in a psychodrama, Calvin was chosen. I felt kind of bad asking him to be my father who molested me when I was little. But he was so much like the good part of my father that I think by choosing Calvin, I was more able to see those good parts.

Another camper shared this perspective:

> Calvin offered such special talents and caring at camp. I guess most people remember how he did "fix-it" things, but what I remember is Calvin and the annual camp hike. Each Free University, Calvin led adults and children out into the forest that surrounds Camp Loma for a full-day hike. Not only did he show us the beauty of the land surrounding camp, he also got us to use our muscles and helped us let go of the emotional intensity of camp. He led those hikes almost to the end of his life.

Another camper said:

> My favorite memory of Calvin is his relationship with his youngest grandchild, Mickey. Calvin had such great love for children, and it just shined through when he was sitting with Mickey, listening to his stories or just holding him when he was upset.

Another camper recalled:

> For many years, Calvin and Marnie were mainstays of camp. They faithfully attended camp year after year, participated on the Committee, and over the years opened their large and lovely home to the many camp families who traveled through northern California. As sfc marked its twenty-fifth year, it also watched Calvin enter into the decline of his life. Although Calvin's physical abilities were not significantly affected by age, his mental capacities began to decline, and soon that decline became quite apparent at camp.
>
> I became fully aware of Calvin's growing disability during the first Temperature Reading at camp several years ago. Marnie and I had been talking about his increasing inability to remember. The memory loss was a struggle for Marnie because Calvin often held Marnie responsible for things caused by his declining memory. In this instance, Calvin could not find a hat that he wanted to give Eliana to use at the opening of Temperature Reading. Marnie repeatedly explained to him that she had given him the hat at breakfast. It was obvious that Calvin had misplaced it between breakfast and Temperature Reading, yet Calvin insisted that Marnie had not given it to him, contending that she probably did not even bring it to camp. When Eliana got up to talk about the Self-esteem Kit and brought out Calvin's hat to use as the detective hat, I thought Marnie would jump out of her seat.
>
> After Temperature Reading, Calvin and Marnie talked about the hat with Eliana. Eliana gently told Calvin that he had given her the hat at breakfast. Even then, I could tell that Calvin was not taking in that he had totally forgotten he had not only had the hat but had given it to Eliana. Eliana was so wonderful with both Calvin and Marnie. She helped them begin a dialogue about Calvin's increasing forgetfulness and the likelihood that it was going to increase. I could tell that Calvin had great difficulty either understanding or accepting—I never could decide which—what Eliana was saying. But his trust in Eliana was so enduring that at least for the moment he was able to acknowledge that he had a problem, which I think lifted a huge burden off Marnie.

During the next year, Calvin's physical health began to decline rapidly, and he was diagnosed with cancer. Within several months of that diagnosis, he died at home. Calvin's final illness and death were quite similar to the way Virginia died. Both were diagnosed with incurable cancer, both chose not to seek advanced medical intervention, and both died at home, surrounded by friends and families. In Calvin's case, all six children, his sisters, members of sfc, and his beloved therapist, Eliana, were able to visit with him immediately before his death.

Sadly, two years later, the SFC community also lost its beloved senior camper, Alicia. [See picture 17 in the section before Part Two]. Alicia came to camp in her early 70s and died just months short of age 93. When interviewed for this book, she talked about how her life changed when she came to camp:

> When I got married, I was 20 years old and believed that once you got married, you stayed married. So I lived for years with a man who was an alcoholic and not much of a husband. By the time he turned 65, I knew I had to live my life; and when he disappointed me one more time, I just left him.
>
> It was very hard to start my life over, so when I heard about camp from a friend I worked with at the local mental health center, I decided to go and see what it was about. I think I was looking for a new family that would support me in my new life. And that is what I got. After I came the first year, I never stopped coming. I love learning about life and how others have coped with different situations. I have learned so much here. I know that I am not alone and that others have faced the same problems I have. I always learn from other people at camp. I'm just stunned to see how camp helps people make changes in their lives.

How I Became a Grandma at Camp

A few years before her death, Alicia shared the following story.

> I think one of the best things that happened to me at camp was the year that Sammy asked me to be his grandma. I have daughters and grandchildren, but somehow the connection I made with this little boy has been so special. I always liked Sammy. He was a terror when he was little, but that is what I liked most: his spunk and curiosity. You could just tell how much he loved camp and the freedom he had to run around and explore and, well, you know, just be a kid. And then, when he was about six or seven, I think, he came to camp and just seemed sad and kind of lost. Right after camp, I ran into him on the way to the latrine, and I asked him if he was sad. He just looked up at me with those wonderful eyes and said, "Can you be my grandma? My grandma died this year, and I need a grandma."
>
> You know, I thought I would just burst into tears, but instead I just put my arms around him and gave him a big hug and said, "You bet. I would be so honored to be your grandma."
>
> And to this day, I feel this special tie with that young man. He has grown up to be a wonderful person, and I feel so proud to have been a part of his life. This is what camp gives each of us: a family that

supports and cares for us throughout our lives, especially when we have lost that, or maybe never had it, in our own families.

Members of the Committee as well as the camp community attended both Calvin's and Alicia's funerals. With the loss of these two enduring members, the SFC community entered a new phase: having to deal with an immediate family's grief and loss as well as the community's loss. Satir Family Camp has now added a new activity, in which the community gathers to remember and memorialize members when they die.

These two deaths also signify how the camp dynamics are changing. For many, it seemed that all camp members would be with the community forever. Yet, just as the children are growing up and attending camp less and less often as their lives became more demanding, the adults are finding themselves facing retirement and the reality that no one can be at camp forever.

Camp Demographics

Like society as a whole, the SFC community is graying. In contrast to years past, children under age 5 are now the smallest group of campers, while applicants over age 45 have increased each year. Teens and young adults are the now largest group of young people in camp. With few exceptions, the young adults came to camp as children and continue to attend with their parents. Committee membership is also made up of older campers who are rapidly reaching retirement age.

These changes in demographics have serious implications for the camp's future. Many of the campers interviewed for this book reported that their children's attachment to camp is what cemented their connection. At times, parents told us, they personally did not want to continue to return to camp, either because their interests had changed or they were not pleased with their experience. Their children insisted that they return. As one father and long-time camper recounted:

> For several years, I wanted to do something different. I do not get that much vacation, and to take one full week for camp just shut off other things I wanted to do with my family. Nevertheless, each year when I suggested that we go somewhere else or just stay home together, the kids voted me down. There was no way they were not coming to camp. Now that they are heading off to college, camp has become the one time of the year when we are all together in one place for a whole week.

A mother of three young adult campers said:

> My kids live all over the country. We keep in contact by e-mail and phone, but camp is the place where we are a family. It is the most important week of the year.

Without families who have young children attending camp, a risk exists that the enduring commitment fostered by the children and then cemented among the long-term campers may not be recreated in the future. The community's aging population also affects how camp functions. Campers over age 70 are exempted from mandatory jobs, and the community is developing ways to meet their needs for more user-friendly camping. To date, these adjustments have included providing assistance in pitching tents, reserving campsites nearer to the facilities, and amplifying work sessions for those with hearing limitations. At Camp Loma, however, only so many adjustments can be made. Inevitably, age and physical impairments will force more campers to leave the community.

Camp Membership

At this point in its development, sfc must decide how to recruit new members. The present plan rests with the offspring of current campers. Three members of that generation have begun families and are bringing their children, the third generation, to camp. However, most of the young adults are just beginning to move from college to employment, which makes it unlikely that this shift in leadership will occur in the immediate future. Awareness is growing in the group that the future of sfc depends on the continued involvement of these young adults as they become more settled in their lives.

Meanwhile, sfc continues to face the challenge of recruiting new families from the larger community. Not surprisingly, the Committee is reluctant to recruit new campers through public venues. As discussed earlier, not all people drawn to a community like sfc can benefit from the camp experience. People who have not had experience with or used mental health services could be overwhelmed by the intensity of the therapeutic experiences that occur at camp. Also, *sfc* is a community that depends on trust. People share very private and personal information at camp, and the depth of that sharing makes all participants vulnerable to each other. Someone who is totally unknown to the community could manipulate, disrupt, or injure others emotionally.

Given all this, sfc has learned that community members have the best sense of who will both benefit from and add to the camp community. Although it is not a fail-safe process for finding appropriate new participants, it has been more successful than not.

Applicants for camp are referred by current campers or by the camp therapists. Both the referring camper and the applicant write a letter to the Committee. Applicants describe themselves, their families, and their reasons for wanting to attend camp. Referring campers also write about each applicant's family, their connection, and what they believe the new family can add to the camp community. The camp registrar is the first person to review the applications and often calls new families to tell them more about camp and to obtain more information. Members of the Committee may raise questions when they review the application and ask the registrar to recontact the family before extending an invitation.

Organizational Issues

Membership is only one of the significant challenges facing sfc. Another is the way it is organized and governed. The Committee continues to be nonhierarchical in structure and makes decisions via process and consensus. When processing issues are fraught with conflict and emotions, effective governance can be difficult. The community has its biggest struggle when passionate speakers sway the group, dominate the process, and contribute to basing decisions on emotions rather than reason. Following these situations, the Committee usually realizes that it needs to rethink its position. Although this ability to reexamine issues is a part of the organization's strength, knowing what is and is not policy often becomes difficult. Ironically, the organization's commitment to Virginia's belief in a nonhierarchical community sometimes limits its effectiveness. As one long-time camper said, "I know I can't be on the Committee. I love camp, I'm committed to its success, and I think I have something to offer, but one Committee meeting, and I'm ready to throttle most of the people there." Even a Committee member and retired manager spoke of drawbacks:

> The Committee both fascinates me and sometimes drives me
> nuts. I have examined all of its decisions and policies back to 1986 and
> found the same issues discussed over and over. The group makes a
> decision, establishes a policy, and then the issue comes up again.
> Someone will say, "Didn't we make a policy about that?" and
> someone (who wants a different policy) will say, "No," and that is the

end of the first policy! The Committee just does its process all over again, makes a new policy, and you watch—in another year or two, the same issue will come up and the same thing will happen again.

This process so frustrates many members with strong organizational skills that they are unwilling to participate on the Committee. At the same time, sfc has now operated successfully for over a quarter of a century. The risk remains, however, that the group will become divided one day, and rather than a few people opting not to participate, the organization itself will not be able to function.

The Camp President

In this type of organization, the president can be the key to how well the Committee functions. That officer is responsible for keeping the group focused and functioning throughout the year as well as during the week at camp. How the president leads and is supported by the other members of the Committee depends a great deal on the individual's personal qualities, experience at camp, and skills as a group leader. How the Committee leader controls or does not control the meeting's process affects the meeting's outcome greatly. Helping the group conduct its discussion and then make a decision is critical to the organization's success. When the group leader is ineffective, the member or members who speak the fastest and the loudest can dominate the process. Even with a weak leader, members of the group can provide facilitation and monitor the process to make sure the group reaches the best decision. However, it is still the president who ensures that people remember and implement the group decisions throughout the year.

Successful leaders have the skills needed to keep sfc focused on its goals and mission and those who understand that mission and remain objective and focused even when tempers and emotions flare, including their own. Because sfc depends on volunteers willing to give generously, of time and sometimes money, not a large group exists from which to select someone with these qualities. It is not surprising, then, that sfc has been content to let an effective leader continue as president for as long as he or she is willing.

Governance and the Next Generation

As the first generation's influence in camp changes and most likely lessens, the camp's original purpose as well as its traditions will likely be affected. Since sfc is no longer a "wilderness camp," the community has already modified policies and traditions that were easier to maintain in a more isolated community. Electronic devices that did not exist during the Pico Blanco years are present in camp, although restricted to individual tents. Cell phone service has improved enough that people can place cell phone calls near camp. Easy access to cars and roads means that campers tend to make trips into town throughout the week. Although debated endlessly by the Committee, the mandate that families arrive on opening day and stay until the end of camp has also eroded. This is particularly true for the younger generation, whose needs prevent attending a full week. By allowing youth (and adults as well) to come to camp for only part of the week, the Committee—many of whom have offspring with demanding schedules—has chosen flexibility over rigid adherence to policies set up in another time and for another type of camp.

Some of the youth who may one day govern sfc are experiencing a camp that differs in many significant ways from the one designed by Virginia Satir. These changes' implications for the community as a whole, however, is not yet fully understood.

Another possible change will be the way the second generation organizes the camp's therapeutic program. When the first generation leaves sfc, it is hard to predict how much of Virginia and her methods will remain in the program. The succeeding generation grew up at camp. Few, if any, of them were at camp or can remember when Virginia led camp. They did not choose to come to camp as adults seeking the experience of this particular type of intentional community. Although it is hoped that the young adults will experience the power of Virginia's work in their own lives and those of their friends, it is not a guarantee. In fact, some young adults attend only their own group sessions and avoid the adult work sessions. They share with each other but have been reluctant to try the more experiential therapy used in the adult sessions. Children who grew up during their camp years are also among those most frustrated by Temperature Reading. One could envision a Committee comprised of these campers ending Temperature Reading because it has been the bane of their existence for decades.

Diversity

An additional issue related to both recruitment and the future of camp is some camp members' longstanding concern about the community's lack of ethnic, racial, and socio-economic diversity. With few exceptions, campers come from white, middle- or upper-middle–class backgrounds. Some diversity does exist within that: families headed by lesbian couples, single parents (both mothers and fathers), families formed through adoption, as well as blended families. However, the camp has never successfully recruited campers from different ethnic, racial, or class groups.

Irrespective of cultural background, sfc's type of therapy focuses on the common human experience. Many members of sfc believe that diversity would add to the effectiveness of camp. The intentional community would gain a certain richness by having more members from different cultures and races living together in this human experiment. However, it has been unsuccessful in meeting that goal. One Latino camper remarked:

> I think one of the challenges for sfc is creating an environment where people from different backgrounds will feel comfortable. Let's face it, this is a pretty white group, and that fact alone makes recruiting people who are not white a challenge.

Another long-time camper pointed out:

> On the one hand, the Committee says it is committed to the concept of diversity. It insists that the camp is open to applicants from all backgrounds. But then it does nothing to specifically recruit people of color. It is going to take more than just saying we want diversity to achieve diversity.

As of the writing of this book, the sfc organization has not addressed this issue. Instead, therapists committed to enriching the community's diversity have recruited the camp's few minority members.

Community Implications

In planning for the future, the Committee is concerned about how to involve young adults in camp governance and leadership. For the camp to survive, the Committee knows that the young adults have to take ownership of the camp's philosophy and provide stewardship in the coming years. To facilitate their involvement, the Committee has accommodated them and works very hard to maintain the status quo. As a result, the community has not had to challenge the current balance, and it remains in the stage of Ennui. This is a time when the community enjoys success, identifies new challenges, and philosophizes about future.

At the same time, the Committee seems reluctant to address the New Status Quo, when abundant energy diversifies to allow individuals more time for questioning and debating the existing structure. Rather, the Committee allows more and more exceptions to the camp's original philosophy and structure—such as electronics at camp, shorter stays, and travel back and forth to town—which forestalls campers from insisting that change occur.

Insistence on change would become the Foreign Element energy. Chaos would follow that, which then fuels Rebellion. Rebellion would require the community to identify its unmet needs and redefine the structure. As much as the Committee states that it wants to address the future, it also struggles to engage in the change process.

To address the future, the community must recruit new families with young children as well as involve the young adults in camp governance. Taking these actions means disrupting the status quo. The Committee's struggle to do so may also perpetuate the stagnation that they currently fear will ultimately be the end of the camp.

Where does Satir Family Camp go from here? Community development is cyclical and folds back into itself over and over, based on members' needs. To continue growing and developing, a community must be challenged with disagreement. Working hard to accommodate everyone can so obscure the community's original purpose as to lose its true mission. It must then return to the Definition stage. For the sfc community to continue developing, the Committee cannot remain invested in maintaining the new status quo. Even at the risk of Chaos and Rebellion, the Committee must allow the change process to occur.

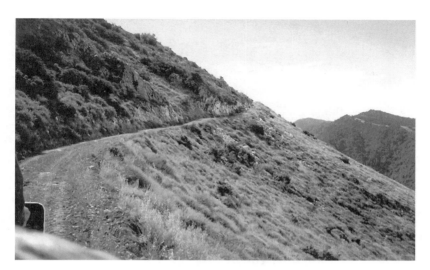

Photo 1.   Road to Pico Blanco

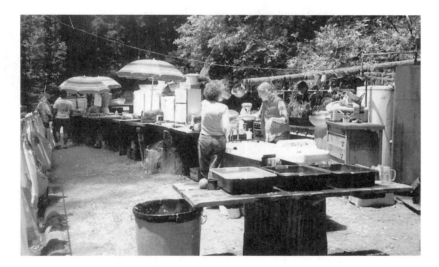

Photo 2.   Pico Blanco kitchen area

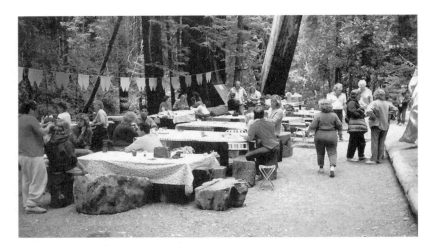

Photo 3.   Pico Blanco eating area

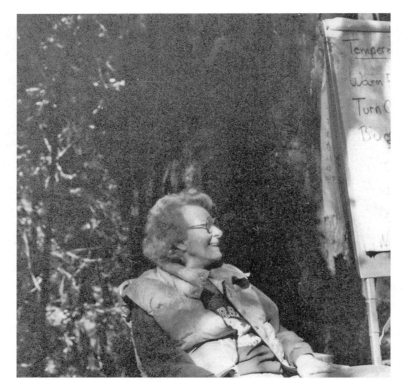

Photo 4.   Virginia at Pico Blanco

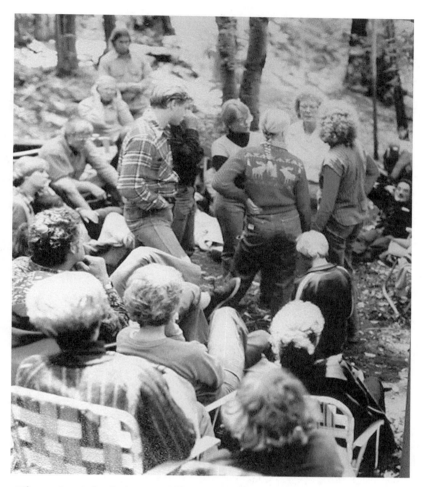

Photo 5.   Virginia conducting a work session

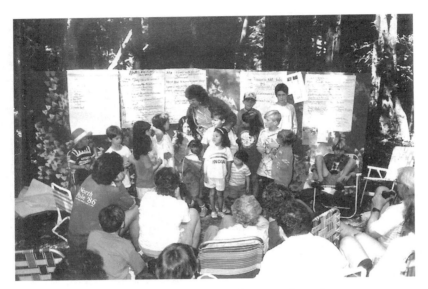

Photo 6.   Children at a work session at Pico Blanco

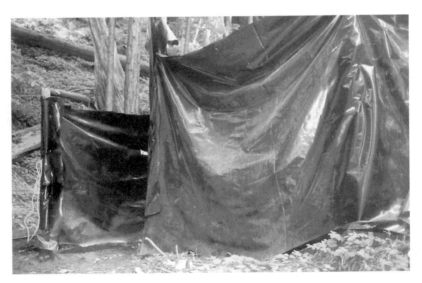

Photo 7.   Outdoor latrine at Pico Blanco

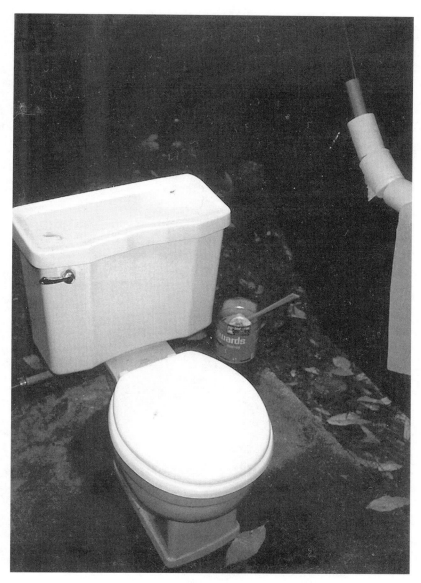

Photo 8.   Pico Blanco latrine

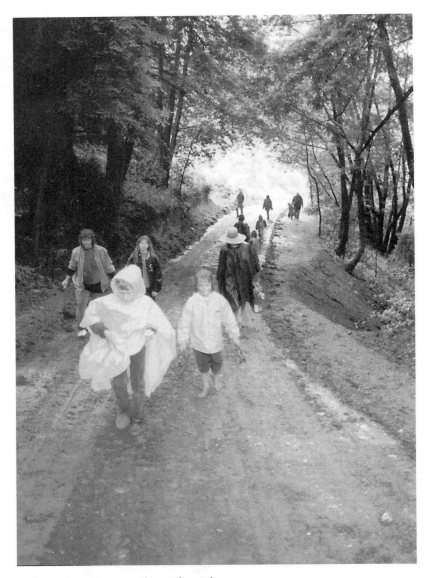

Photo 9.   Evacuating Pico Blanco

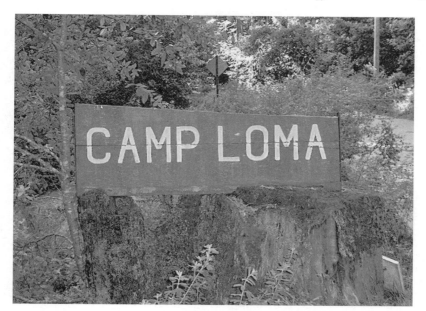

Photo 10.   Entrance to Camp Loma

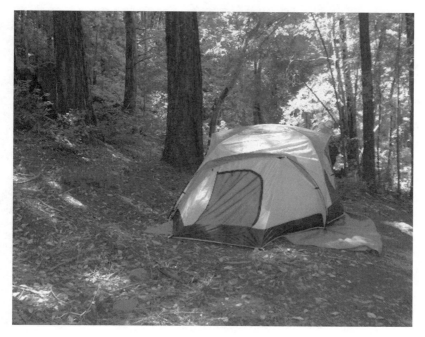

Photo 11.   Camp Loma campsite

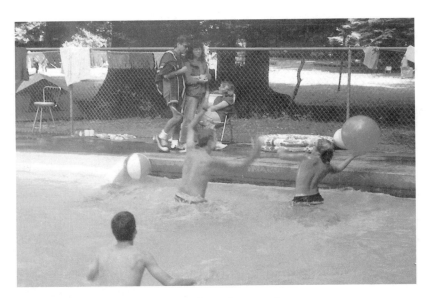

Photo 12.   Camp Loma swimming pool

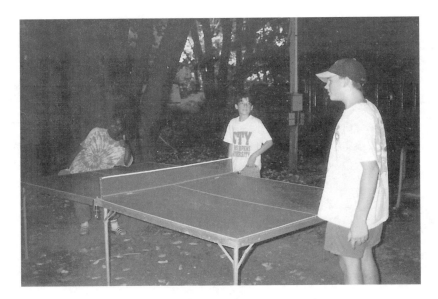

Photo 13.   Playing ping pong at Camp Loma

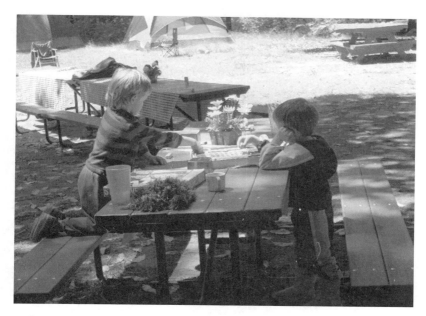

Photo 14.   Playing board games at Camp Loma

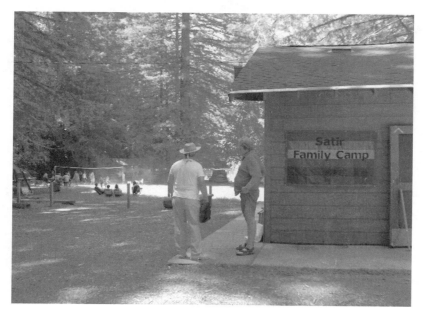

Photo 15.   Free time at Camp Loma

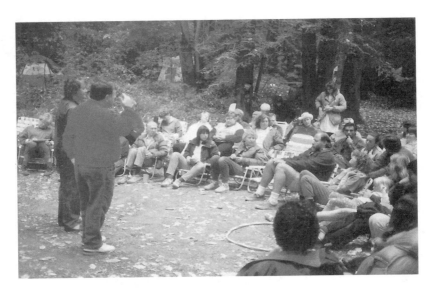

Photo 16.   A work session at Camp Loma

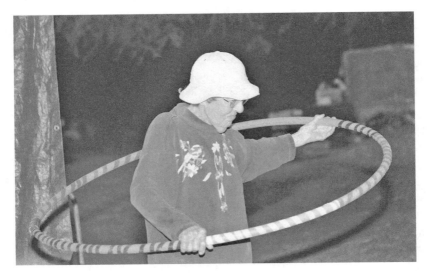

Photo 17.   Senior SFC camper at play

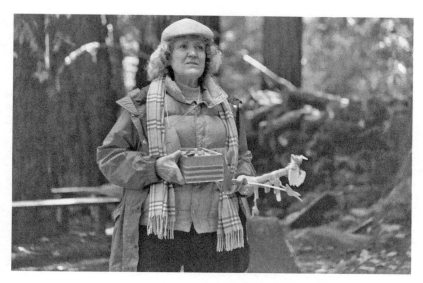

Photo 18.   Laura Dodson presenting Self-Esteem Kit

Photographers

Photo 1	Liv Monroe
Photos 2–6	Virginia Satir Archives
Photos 7–9	Liv Monroe
Photos 10, 11	Elsa Ten Broeck
Photos 12, 13	Liv Monroe
Photos 14, 15	Bob Bonar
Photo 16	Liv Monroe
Photos 17, 18	Bob Bonar

Part Two

Adaptation of Satir Principles and Methods at Family Camp

The therapy program is a key way that sFC maintains Virginia's legacy. Each work session teaches camp members about Virginia's theories and methods. The work sessions also contribute to the development of lifetime bonds among members of the community. As one therapist said:

> There are many different reasons and ways that intentional communities are created. To be successful over the years, it is important that there be a unifying theme or reason to keep people connected to that community. In my opinion, the therapeutic work we do at sFC has made this community unique, because the work fosters deep and life-long connections between people. As people share their lives and their innermost feelings, they develop bonds that maintain their connections even when the community is faced with crises, as all communities must face. This type of community is not for everyone, but for the people who are willing to open themselves to the depth of connections that are made here, it is truly magical.

We wrote Part Two to help the reader understand how that magic develops. We discuss the Satir principles that underpin the community and guide the therapy program. This part of the book also presents Satir methods, techniques, and therapeutic strategies that have been adapted to an intentional community setting and/or used in family, individual, or group work. Finally, Part Two provides two examples of Satir methods used at sFC.

8

Satir Principles, Theories, and Methods

The following principles, all taken from Virginia's written words (Loeschen, 1991), form the philosophical underpinnings of the Satir Family Camp's intentional community.

Satir Principles

In all of her work with individuals, families, and groups, Virginia Satir used these guiding principles:

We are all manifestations of life.
We are all equal in value.
We are all unique.
We are born perfect with everything within us. We have the resources we need.
Self-esteem is a birthright for everyone.
Communication is to relationships as breath is to life.
We are not our feelings. Feelings belong to us. We are in charge of our feelings.
Feelings we have in the present are often generated by thoughts from the past.
The only real certainty in life is change.
People are capable of change.
There is more pull toward the familiar than the unfamiliar.
The problem is not the problem, the coping is the problem.

We cannot change the events of the past, but we can change
our coping when it is no longer useful.
Transformation has occurred when we go from saying, "I want
to be loved" to "I am loved—by me."

From this foundation, Virginia helped people create a more
satisfying life and become more fully human.

Satir Theories

As discussed in Chapter 2, Virginia's personal experiences with
psychoanalysis affected her professional work. She came away determined to use her skills and wisdom to help people in a different way,
avoiding techniques or theories that viewed people seeking mental
health services as suffering from pathology. During that quest, she
developed theories about human development that described people's
behavior as responses to early life struggles that were necessary to
assure survival. She also believed that people eventually need to
change many of their early survival behaviors when they no longer
served their original purpose. Virginia's unlimited sense of optimism
about the human condition underlies all her theories about human
behavior. She fervently believed that all humans are capable of learning, making choices, and ultimately making changes in their behavior. We discuss two of her primary theories that underlie many of the
premises and much of the work done at sfc.

Human Growth Model

In her Human Growth Model, Virginia describes how people
relate, view the world, and view change (Satir et al., 1991, pp. 14, 15).
The model states that every individual is unique and is defined from
an inner source of strength and validation rather than by external
measurements. Further, all individuals are equal to all other individuals in the world. Roles and status exist only within specific contexts
and do not determine a person's total identity. Change is an ongoing
life process that occurs from the cellular to the cosmic level and provides individuals with opportunities to move into new areas and discover options that may not have been available without change. Using
this theory as her prism, Virginia helped each client see his or her
value and equality in a world that may have left that person behind
or run roughshod over him or her. She believed that as people became

"more fully human" they would recognize their inherent worth and place in the world (Satir et al., 1991, pp. 85–119).

Virginia created sfc as a place for her to explore how a group of unrelated families living together in the wilderness for one week per year would create a community using the principles of the Human Growth Model. By design, the sfc community is a nonhierarchical community in which all persons in camp are equal participants in the organization. Campers come together to foster the human growth of all members. At camp, community members are able to try on new roles and to develop or refine their identities. The story of the "Collapsing Camper" in Chapter 5 is an example of a community member trying on new roles and identities while at camp. All members work diligently to understand their interaction with others within the camp and to use the camp experience to increase their understanding of how they relate to others outside of camp.

Human Validation Process Model

In family therapy, Virginia worked from a place of health and transformation rather than pathology and symptoms. In The Human Validation Process Model, Virginia redefines "symptoms" as "blocked energy" that can be reshaped and transformed into a useful purpose. What other practitioners considered the "presenting symptom," Virginia viewed as positive energy that helped people survive in negative environments. She postulated that when the need for that energy ("symptom") was altered, the energy could either be transformed or eliminated. In the Human Validation Process Model, Virginia also stated that, except for genetic endowment, which is set at birth, a person's feelings, thoughts, and behaviors are all the direct result of learning that occurs during early childhood. Therefore, any person who chooses to can also relearn those behaviors and ultimately change his or her behavior. The therapeutic techniques used at sfc reflect this theory of human behavior. The camp uses the techniques that Virginia developed to address defenses and coping methods (resulting from early childhood learning, traumas, or confusion) that cause people to cut off or disown parts of themselves. Helping adults and children deal with the wounds of early childhood is one of the great gifts that the sfc therapeutic program gives its members.

As described in campers' comments and stories throughout this book, relationships in camp often mirrored the dysfunction and challenges community members faced in their lives outside of camp. Not all members of camp like or respond well to each other. Jealousies and rivalries exist, and some members are simply challenging to live with. As a result, daily life at camp often becomes the grist that helps campers both experience and examine how they relate to others. Some of the techniques described in this chapter demonstrate therapeutic work that focuses on the relationships between campers. Some demonstrate the therapeutic work of campers who struggle with growth issues in their lives outside camp. And, sometimes, as one might expect, the two become intermingled until the outside stressors are so tied to relationships and events within camp that they are virtually indistinguishable.

Satir Techniques*

Virginia's techniques help "make the implicit explicit, the unfamiliar familiar, and the unexpressed expressed in order to develop new awareness" (Satir & Baldwin, 1983, p. 239). Therapists at sfc use Virginia's creative techniques to teach and demonstrate her principles and theories about human development, communication, families, and communities. The concepts and skills that therapists teach during the work sessions are applied throughout the week to help the community grow, develop and, when necessary, survive its challenges. Work done by individuals often creates issues within the community, which create growth not just for individuals but for the community at large. Consider the alcohol and drug issue explored over the years at camp and discussed in Chapter 4. Family struggles with teenage drinking as well as individual and family struggles with sobriety become mirrored in camp life. Fortunately, sfc provides the opportunity, techniques, and support to work through the challenges that occur in all aspects of life, both at camp and in the outside world.

Although Virginia developed many techniques that continue to be used in traditional family therapy, sfc focuses on a few techniques that adapt well to a communal camp setting. These techniques include:

Process
Temperature Reading
Self-Esteem Tool Kit
Work Sessions

---

*To learn more about Satir methods, we encourage people to read *The Satir Model* (Satir, Banmen, Gerber, & Gomori, 1991) and *Satir Step by Step* (Satir & Baldwin, 1983).

Metaphor
Drama
Sculpture
Parts Party
Family Reconstruction

Process

By far the most powerful technique used at sfc is "process." As Millman (1995, p. 25) says in "The Law of Process: Taking Life Step by Step":

Process transforms any journey
into a series of small steps,
taken one by one,
to reach any goal.
Process transcends time,
teaches patience,
rests on a solid foundation
of careful preparation,
and embodies trust
in our unfolding potential.

Process, as described in the preceding poem, applies to both an individual's inner experience as well as to external experiences that occur in a group. *Internal process* examines a person's feelings, the meanings he or she gives to those feelings, the feelings about the emotions being examined, and the internal yearnings that create the feelings (Satir et al., 1991, p. 157). *Group process* describes the external interactions that occur among people. Group process focuses on the way a group reaches a goal or a decision rather than on the outcome. Group process emphasizes the importance of each group member and focuses on obtaining group input to assure that any decision or goal both considers and reflects the opinions and needs of the entire group. All Satir-based work uses both of these tools frequently. To understand Satir Family Camp, it is important to understand how process is a tool and an end result.

Satir Family Camp refers to itself as a process community. As such, the community is both committed to and utilizes group and individual internal process to address any member or group of members' concerns, ideas, issues, experiences, and expectations. Through the consistent use of group and individual process, sfc builds and enhances interdependence and caring among its members and provides a model of solving problems and resolving conflict. The entire camp relies heavily on individual and group process to stimulate the community's development. The purest form of process used at sfc is found in Temperature Reading.

Temperature Reading

Virginia developed Temperature Reading to help groups improve their communication and self-esteem. She chose the name as a metaphor for measuring an individual's as well as a group's internal and external environment. Temperature Reading helps assess, change, or maintain an individual's or a group's "temperature." Temperature Reading is the only mandatory activity at sfc. It begins each camp day and is the time when structured group processing occurs. The technique encourages everyone who has a concern, an observation, a thought, or an idea related to an issue raised during Temperature Reading to raise his or her voice. By stressing process over outcome, sfc reinforces the value of all points of view and concerns as well as each individual's value in the community. By taking the time and getting broad input, the community addresses most concerns. Decisions, when needed, are reached by consensus. Temperature Reading is thus one manifestation of Virginia's Human Growth Model.

Temperature Reading includes discussion of: "Appreciations," "Bugs" (complaints) or "Puzzles," "New Information," and "Hopes and Wishes." All members, from the eldest to the youngest, have time both to speak and be heard regarding any issue they wish to bring to the community's attention. The guidelines for a Temperature Reading are:

1. All members are expected to attend.
2. Everyone may speak.
3. When someone reports a bug, that person is also asked to provide a solution or recommendation to deal with the bug.

Temperature Reading reinforces equality in the group by giving each person equal stature, responsibility, and voice in the community.

"Appreciations" generally go like this:

Nadine [*a new camper*]: My name is Nadine. I want to thank Lois and Stefan for inviting me to camp. I feel very lucky to be here and part of this amazing group of people. I have been hoping to find a community where I feel both welcome and at home. I have been here for two days and feel that I have found that place. Thank you, Lois and Stefan, for making this possible.

Susie [*age 4, amid giggles*]: I want to thank Jacob and Lucinda for wanting to come to camp 'cause they brought Jamie, and now I have someone to play with.

Nita [*a camp facilitator*]: I want to thank Rich and Glen for picking us up at the airport and helping us get all our stuff from baggage claim to the car and then into our campsite. You made my adjustment to being back in the woods much smoother.

"Bugs" generally increase as the week goes by. Some Bugs return year after year.

Paulie [*age 10*]: I have a bug about the games. Last night, I was playing chess and made certain that I put away all the pieces when I finished. Today, I went back to play another game, and the king and the queen are missing. My solution is that anyone who plays with a game needs to put back all the pieces, and if they are too little to do that, then they are too little to be playing with the game. [*This last sentence is addressed to his younger brother Samuel, who comes up to him and hands over the king and queen*].

Katlin: Last night, there was music and loud noises coming from the dining area well after 10 p.m. I know the games were fun, but I really need to sleep if I am going to be able to take care of the twins all day. My suggestion is that everyone remembers the 10 p.m. lights out and respect the rule that noise should also cease or at least be reduced after 10 p.m.

The next part of Temperature Reading, "New Information," communicates announcements, changes in schedules, reminders, upcoming events, and so on. Depending on the events that are occurring on a particular day, this portion can become very lengthy. When possible, people use humor to lessen the boredom. Additionally, as in the example below, it also serves to help the group's youngest members to recognize their worth in facilitating the community's process.

Temperature Reading leader: Before we begin New
Information, who has a joke? Leo—where is Leo?

Leo [*age 6 and king of the "Knock Knock" jokes*]: Knock, knock.

Camp: Who's there?

Leo: Doncha.

Camp: Doncha who?

Leo: Doncha wish Temperature Reading was over right now?!!

However, Temperature Reading does not end until all campers
have an opportunity to share their "Hopes and Wishes" for the day.
Many are mundane, such as the universal lost object;

Alta: I have a hope and wish that the book I was reading, Sue
Grafton's *O Is for Outlaw,* will be found and put on Pico
Junko [*the table where lost items gather to wait for their owners
to discover them*].

Lucy: I have a hope and wish that someone will switch lunch
cleanup with me so that I can go to the children's group
with Randy. He wants to make a plate and asked me if I
would help him make it.

Other hopes or wishes can result in a change in schedule to accommodate the needs of individuals or groups that arise during the
week.

Lincoln: A number of issues have come up this week about
teens and their involvement in camp. I have a hope and a
wish that we can take an afternoon work session and have
a joint meeting with the teen group to talk about how we
can come together as a community.

Many discussions that begin at Temperature Reading are critical
to the community's growth. At the same time, the processing that goes
on often results in protracted discussions and very long meetings. The
annual sfc evaluations consistently show that Temperature Reading is
the least popular activity. For children, the experience is a huge bore
because they have to sit and listen to an endless amount of adult talk.
Teenagers are usually frustrated at the adults' need to "talk everything
to death." Many adults share this frustration. Usually, sometime during the week, discussion arises about how to reduce the time spent in

Temperature Reading. At that point, the following phrase never fails to surface: "Trust the process."

If a community is going to grow and thrive, Virginia knew that its members must have a place and time that allows and encourages everyone to communicate his or her feelings. Without this, the demands and stresses of community life, particularly an intense environment such as camp, could lead to the community's destruction.

Virginia had a particular interest in children learning that they have a voice equal to and as important as any adult voice. Temperature Reading is the place where sfc children, often at a very young age, learn to speak their needs, feelings, and opinions to the community at large. Throughout the week, facilitators also encourage children to speak in their family groups, community meetings, or therapeutic groups.

Temperature Reading can also work in group and family therapy settings. Using this technique at the beginning of a session helps everyone achieve an equal voice and gain insight into each other's starting point. For instance, Hopes and Wishes can help identify issues members want to work on in the session. Likewise, Bugs is a great place to outline the work for the session as well as a way to bring out conflict. Finally, Appreciations can provide the format for practicing appropriate social skills in a group setting, and it can help family members recognize and acknowledge the love and respect they have for each other.

Self-Esteem Kit

Each year, generally at the first Temperature Reading, an sfc therapist introduces all members of camp to Virginia's therapeutic tool called the "Self-Esteem Kit." Using props (developed by a camp member) to illustrate each concept, the therapist teaches even the youngest camp members about Virginia's belief that each person has everything he or she needs to survive, grow, and challenge life. The Self-Esteem Kit is a simple but powerful metaphor that explains how all people have and can enhance the self-esteem needed to become more fully human. The following poem, written by Virginia (in Satir et al., 1991, p. 298), aptly describes the importance of being fully human.

To Be More Fully Me
I need to remember

I am me
And in all the world there is no one like me.
I give myself permission
To discover me and use me
Lovingly.
I look at myself and see
A beautiful instrument
In which that can happen.
I love me, I appreciate me,
I value me.

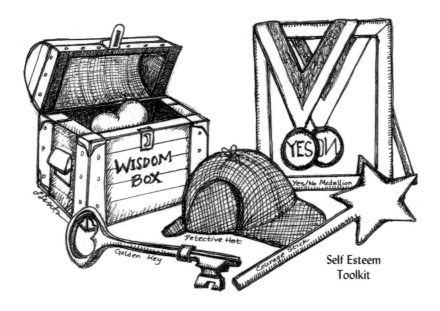

The Self-Esteem Tool Kit has five elements:

1. Detective Hat
2. Yes/No Medallion
3. Courage Stick (also called an Empowering and Wishing
   Wand)
4. Golden Key
5. Wisdom Box

Virginia described the Kit in the following meditation (in Satir et al., 1991, pp. 296–97).

> The first thing in this kit is a detective hat, which you put on immediately when there is a puzzle or a question or an effort to understand: How do the pieces fit together? How do you explore for the gaps and find the things that fit? This is in contrast to judging. Many people judge before they explore, but I would like to recommend to you that you keep your detective hat handy for any time a question, puzzle or gap appears, so you can go on a journey of exploration.
>
> The second thing in your kit is a medallion that you can hang around your neck. On one side in beautiful jeweled letters, it says, "YES." Underneath that "YES" it says, "Thank you for noticing me. What you ask of me at this time fits just fine. The answer is yes."
>
> And on the other side in equally beautiful jeweled letters the word "NO." Underneath that is says, "Thank you for noticing me. What you ask of me at this time doesn't fit at all. The answer is no."
>
> This is the key to your integrity. Yes and No are both loving words. When you say yes and you feel no, or when you say no and you feel yes, you have eroded your integrity and weakened yourself. So keep your medallion fresh within your awareness, and always say the real yes and the real no, keeping your integrity intact and keeping your strength strong.
>
> The next thing in the kit is an Empowering Wand, a Courage Stick, a Wishing Wand—all three. All three names can stand for the same thing. And when you feel a wish or a desire to move in a direction, you can take this empowering wand in your hand and move, dragging your fears behind you, if they're there. If you wait until all your fears are taken care of, you probably will never move ahead. As you take that empowering wand, wishing wand, courage stick in your hand and move forward, many times your fear will have been dissolved by the time you reach where you want to go.
>
> . . . The next thing in the kit is a Golden Key. The golden key enables you to open any door to ask any question, to make speakable what is unspeakable, and to attempt to do the undoable—to make it doable—opening up all the possibilities, looking in all the cracks, noticing even the smallest kind of movement. That's your golden key.
>
> The next thing in the kit is a Wisdom Box. The wisdom box is part of your heritage. It's part of what you came into the world with. And for me, I have located it by going into my navel two inches and going up toward my heart. Halfway between, I find the wisdom box.
>
> This wisdom box is in contact with all the wisdom of the universe—all the wisdom of the past and all of that which resides within you. It is that part which you sense sometimes giving direction;

sometimes it's called the still, small voice. It is that part deep inside that knows and that tries to give directions. Like a thought or a feeling, you will not find it on a surgery table. You won't find the wisdom box there, but I don't question the presence of a wisdom box. It is that part of us, when we are cleared of all of our defenses and all our fears, in which we can hear the stirrings of our growth and our wisdom. Perhaps our greatest job in life is to remove all that stands between ourselves and our wisdom, and then to recognize that all human beings have a wisdom box. It needs only to be tapped.

Let yourself now be in touch again with your breathing, and if those tools are not already within your grasp, or you have not already used them, could you give yourself permission to try them on for size and let them become yours?

As you make more use of your wisdom box, and all of your tools, you can go into your psychological closet to examine what is there for you—what you need right now. And you may find that there are things there that came about as a result of your saying yes when you felt no—which might include anger, rage, or resentment. Or you may find things there that have been said to you in the past, "You don't deserve to go farther, you have done bad things." But you will recognize this for what it is: a misunderstanding of you and yourself. And as you clear your closet of these things by sorting them, by noticing them, and by letting them go, you can make room for new things that come as a result of new ways of viewing yourself.

Opportunity for new visions and ways to get there is enhanced by your connection with the center of the Earth, which brings energy upward to your feet and legs and gives groundedness—the ability to think, to know, collect knowledge, and to be reasonable. You are also a recipient of energy from the heavens, which moves downward through your face and neck into your arms and torso, bringing with it the energy of imagination, of intuition, of sensing—the kind of thing that gives color and song and texture to your life.

And as the two come together, they create a third energy—that which allows you to move from the inside of yourself to the outside, where you can connect with those eyes and ears and arms and skin and ideas that are ready and open. For those that are still in bud form, not yet ready, allow yourself to notice, love, and pass by.

So this morning as you come into this day, give yourself permission to know that your underpinnings are solid; that you are a wonderful, magnificent being of this universe, and you have only to learn about that magnificence.

At the beginning of the first Temperature Reading of each camp, facilitators present the Self-Esteem Kit to remind campers about the tools they each have to explore their human journey together. [See the last photo in the section just before Part Two].

The Self-Esteem Kit also works in individual, family, and group therapy. It can be useful when working on issues of passivity and assertion as well as expanding a client's understanding of where other people are coming from in relationships. Because it is a nonthreatening intervention, it can be particularly useful resolving issues between two people in a session and/or in assisting an individual to see other points of view outside the session. Lastly, this technique can provide a metaphor for exploring old messages, identities, and internal conflicts that continue to haunt present relationships.

Work Sessions

Facilitators usually schedule ten sessions per camp, each lasting two to three hours. Trained therapists utilize Satir methods to address the concerns of individuals, couples, families, and small groups. Work sessions are open to all campers, and attendance is voluntary.

SFC therapists adapt Virginia's techniques to fit the community's setting and uniqueness of design. The SFC model is very different from both traditional office therapy and Virginia's Process Communities. At SFC, therapy is the basis of daily life. The intensity of the work sessions spreads into community life removing the distance and boundaries that normally occur between therapy and daily life.

An additional strength of the work-session approach to therapy is the involvement of observers as well as the participant(s). From Virginia's time to the current day, work sessions generate intense and often highly emotional content. Simply attending a work session can increase a person's awareness of his or her own feelings and reactions to the issues addressed at the work sessions. Those who attend often become as involved in the work as the person(s) "doing" the work. To help illustrate and understand the issues being addressed, observers also often participate in psychodramas or sculptures.

Work Session Techniques

Virginia viewed techniques "as a way of engaging in one specific activity to meet the emergent need of a person or a group at that moment" (Satir & Baldwin, 1983, p. 240). Many of her techniques utilize *experimental activities*, which Virginia defined as "activities that maximize participants' learning and ability to use learning for change. . . . New ways of looking at one's own and other's behavior" (*ibid*, p. 240). To implement them effectively, many of these techniques require group participation. These techniques help participants experience the feelings that traditional therapy often simply talks about.

Virginia was ahead of her time in the ways that she applied adult learning principles to therapeutic experiences. By incorporating physicality and visual stimulation into her techniques, she engaged not only the primary participants but also community members who were observing the work. Her experience as a young deaf child probably contributed to her intuitive understanding of the need for physical movement in communication and retention as well as in engaging others through physical touch.

sfc therapists utilize many of Virginia's well-tested and effective techniques, including meditations, metaphors, drama, sculpting, the Parts Party, and Family Reconstruction. The following passages describe each of these in brief, and the next chapter includes examples of a couple of them.

Meditations are a technique Virginia used to help people use the brain's right hemisphere. Meditation helps participants focus their energy, become open to their intuitive nature, quiet their inner "dialogue," and be more fully present in the "now" (Satir et al., 1991, p. 292).

A *metaphor* is a figure of speech in which a word or phrase denotes one kind of object or idea in place of another to suggest a likeness or analogy between them. Metaphors develop awareness by linking two events, ideas, characteristics, or meanings and transforming the experiences from one mode to another. Virginia used metaphors to give information in a nonthreatening manner because they allow a certain distance from the situation. Metaphors also help reinforce learning.

Drama in many forms can help people act out or observe events from a safe distance. Virginia believed that people learned and changed through experiencing feelings, so she used many forms of drama to stimulate this process. As she and Michele Baldwin wrote (1983, p. 246):

> Drama is the expression of internal images, which goes beyond linear expression of words. It provides metaphorical expression of inner states. Drama allows participants to have an opportunity to return to a situation or to know about the life of another person from the inside. It allows the development of new connections with people with whom they relate.

The *sculpting* technique uses participants' bodies—including gestures, closeness or distance, and movement—to reflect family relationships and communication. Sculpting is particularly effective in making past experiences come alive in the present (Satir & Baldwin, 1983, p. 244).

In the *Parts Party*, the goal is to help a person become aware that he or she is made up of many different parts. This technique helps a person become acquainted with, understand, and become aware of how the parts relate to each other. Participants also become aware of their choices about when and how to use these parts. Designed to help people learn how to use all their parts in a more harmonious and integrated manner, this activity helps people become aware of inner resources and find ways to use them more effectively in their present state. Alternatively, they learn how to transform their parts' energy into more useful states, turning them into assets rather than liabilities (*ibid*, p. 258).

As originally designed by Virginia, the Parts Party is a very structured exercise that can require hours of work to prepare and deliver. At sfc, therapists usually adapt this technique into two approaches. In the less structured approach, therapists use the parts to help clarify work that is in progress. The more structured approach uses the Parts Party in the entire work. In either case, therapists must be very skilled and experienced to adapt what is a complicated and lengthy process into the two- or three-hour work session used at camp.

The *Family Reconstruction* exercise helps a person re-experience early feelings and emotions and gain clarity about early childhood from the perspective of an adult rather than a child. Using this technique, a participant becomes aware of how early experiences have affected him or her throughout life. By transforming old coping mechanisms into an adult-based reality, Family Reconstruction also provides new models for living. A fully developed Family Reconstruction also helps the participant look at his or her parents through the eyes and perspective of an adult rather than a child. The goal of a Family Reconstruction is to help the participant act from choice rather than from compulsion (Satir & Baldwin, 1983, pp. 253–58).

In their traditional forms, the preceding techniques require time (both to prepare and deliver) that is simply not available at camp. Therapists at sfc must assess the presenting problem or issue rapidly and decide what therapeutic technique is appropriate for both the individual (or couple, family, or group). Therapists must also be well versed in all the techniques and able to use abbreviated versions.

Working in teams of two or three per session, sfc therapists draw on their combined insight and understanding.

These techniques challenge the idea that a person must be directly engaged in work on an issue to change and grow. Virginia's concept of work sessions demonstrates her belief that individuals can make use of and grow from observing the work of others and from participating in someone else's historical reenactments.

Virginia developed her therapeutic tools over time and often through her life experience, both as a child and an adult. Each technique also stems from her theories and beliefs about both human and community development. One can see connections throughout her theories and techniques to the sad, neglected, precocious child who went deaf between the ages of 2 and 5.

9

Satir Family Camp Therapeutic Techniques

This chapter demonstrates how a Parts Party and a Family Reconstruction might occur at SFC. Both examples are composites of work done at camp.

Alisa's Parts Party

The Parts Party adapts easily to the SFC setting. Therapists can apply it to just part of a work session or can use it as the primary technique, as the following story demonstrates.

Alisa: When I got to camp the year after I retired, I felt so let down and just disappointed with my life. I had worked so hard at camp and in therapy to deal with the effects of being molested, and I thought finally I could live my life as an adult without all that heavy stuff weighing me down. I looked forward to retiring. I had many ideas about what I would do with this newfound freedom. I looked forward to time with myself as well as with Neal, my life partner.

Instead, I found myself doing nothing. So when I got to camp, I went to talk with Glen [*a camp therapist*]. I wasn't sure this issue really warranted a work session. This struggle seemed minor to the struggles most people worked on in camp.

When Glen described his idea of using a Parts Party to help me look at how I was dealing with this phase of my life, I decided it would be a special way to look at the problem and decided to try it.

Glen: Early in the week, Alisa came to me to discuss the struggle she was having now that she was retired. She had left a high-pressure job and was feeling both let down and disappointed with this new phase of her life. Alisa and I had worked together during several previous camps regarding her childhood and had made significant progress integrating those early life experiences. This year, she was dealing with a life change that affected many parts of her life, and I immediately thought about using the Parts Party to address those issues.

Because the time available to do work at camp is limited, therapists often meet to do some preliminary work with the person. This helps maximize time in the work session. Glen met with Alisa to explain the Parts Party technique and to help her begin some preparatory thinking about her issues within the context of the technique. Later, at the work session, Glen began by asking:

Glen: Alisa, can you describe why you decided to work today?

Alisa: Well, I retired last year and things just seem very confusing right now.

Glen: What does "confusing" feel like?

Alisa: Mixed up, unsettled, maybe disappointed.

Glen: Which feels the strongest?

Alisa: Uh, I'm not sure what you mean.

Glen: Well, you described three feelings: mixed up, unsettled, and disappointed. I'm just wondering which feels the strongest right now.

Alisa [*standing silently, beginning to cry, and then saying quietly*]: Disappointed.

Glen [*moving closer*]: Can you tell me what the tears are about?

Alisa: I'm just so sad. I thought being retired would make things better, but all I do is feel sad. [*Her crying increases*].

Glen: So you also feel sad. Are there any other feelings coming up?

Alisa: I guess I'm confused . . . [*She pulls away suddenly and stands straighter with fists clenched*]. No, I feel ripped off. This is not what I want. I should be having fun, and I should be full of energy, and instead I just feel lost and unable to do anything.

Glen: Now I see anger along with the sadness. . . . I also hear many "shoulds."

Alisa: Yeah, I did have expectations, and I am really pissed at how things turned out. Actually, I'm really pissed at myself. Why can't I be as happy as Vince, Sondra, and all the others who are able to retire and not fall apart? Why do I always have to do it so . . . so messed up?!

Glen: More "shoulds": "I should be having fun, I should be relaxed, I should do it the way Vince and Sondra do it." Is there something or someone telling you all those "shoulds"?

Alisa: Well, me, I guess.

Glen [*smiling*]: Yes, it's all you, but is there a particular part of you that is generating those "shoulds"?

Alisa: Well, I know there is a voice in my head that keeps saying, "See, I told you so, I told you the minute you retired, you would just freak out and do nothing 'cause you can't survive without structure." This voice just keeps saying, "You are going to wig out and go totally nuts." And right now, I kind of feel . . . [*Her voice drops off.*]

Glen: Right now you feel . . . ?

Alisa: Like I'm going to totally lose it and just be crazy.

Glen: Well, that would be okay, if you need to. I'm right here to keep you grounded, and you have the whole group to support you, if that is what you need to do.

Alisa: I don't think I really need to do it. I think it's just a fear I have.

Glen: Okay, so what I'm hearing is that you are struggling with this new part of your life, that you have conflicts within yourself about whether you can be a complete person if you are not employed, and that you are afraid that without structure, you may go crazy. How am I doing so far?

Alisa: That sounds like me.

Glen: Earlier in the week, when you told me about this struggle and that you might want to do some work, I suggested that we do a Parts Party to help you sort out the confusion inside. Does that still seem right to you?

Alisa: Yeah, I think I just described some parts while we were talking.

Glen: I agree, so why don't we begin by seeing how many different parts we can identify? [*Turning to Nita, another therapist*]: Nita, can you write these on the paper so we make sure we remember them all?

At this point, Glen moved into the first phase of the Parts Party. He and Alisa have stated the issue, clarified it, and agreed to proceed into the Parts Party.

Glen: What would you call the part that feels like it is going crazy without structure?

Alisa: Uh . . . I guess my Melodramatic Part.

Glen: Can we give the part a name—maybe that of some famous person?

Virginia found that giving parts the names of famous people or names that are important to the participant often adds dimension to the part. The name that the participant chooses often reveals some information about that part.

Alisa: Well, I always felt like, when I get into the drama thing, I feel like Marlene Dietrich.

Glen: Good, Marlene Dietrich it is. How about the part of you that's sad?

Alisa: I need a name?

Glen: Well, let's talk about it, and then if there is a name that fits, we'll add it.

Alisa: This is the part that brings the tears. This is the part that always feels let down and kind of uncared for. Maybe it isn't so much sad as little.

Glen: So, do you think there is a name for this part?

Alisa: I think I'll call her "Little Bit."

Glen: And I heard you talk about a voice that keeps talking to you about your actions and what you are doing. Can you name that voice?

Alisa: Oh, yeah, that's the Judge, yeah, "Judge Judy," no doubt about it.

Glen: Not all the parts have to be women, you know. You could have parts that are the masculine part of you.

Alisa: Okay, but that part is definitely a woman. Kind of my mother, I think.

The process continued as Glen helped Alisa identify, describe, and name the parts of her personality, both conscious and subconscious. Each part illuminates the struggle she was having in this phase of her life. At the end of the discussion, Glen restated the names and descriptions that Nita had recorded on the board at the back of the session area.

Glen: So, let's be sure that we have a list of the parts and the way you described them. Nita put up: Marlene: the melodramatic part that will go crazy without structure; Little Bit: the child part that is always sad because she feels let down and disappointed; Harriet: the elderly part that is unable to do anything. This part is connected to your awareness that you have a family history of Alzheimer's Disease; Eleanor Roosevelt: the retired part that is full of energy, fun, and ideas; Hillary Clinton: the part who functioned at work, was in charge of everything, had respect and high self-esteem; Lolita: the sexually active part that enjoys conquests and sexual relationships but is also childlike in her sexual exploits; Partner: the part that is committed to her partner and domestic stability without sexual energy or passion; Judge Judy: the critical part that is never satisfied and predicts doom at every turn.

Is there anything you want to add or change?

Alisa shook her head, indicating no changes are needed. Glen then entered the second part of the technique, where the person doing the work (whom Virginia called the "Star") provides adjectives for each part and, in that process, adds more depth and meaning to each part.

Glen: Alisa, I want you to look at your list of parts and give me a one-word adjective that describes each one. Nita will write the adjective up beside the name. Is that clear?

Alisa: Not really.

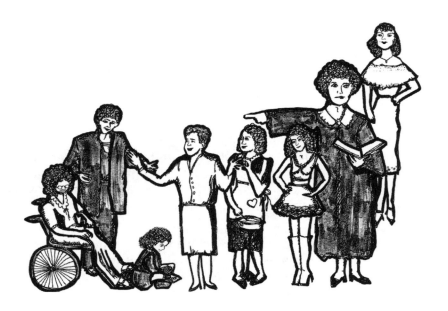

Glen: Okay, let me explain a little more. All the parts that you have identified have particular meaning to you. Virginia created this next part of the exercise to help both you and me better understand the meanings by adding descriptors to the names. How about we start with one or two adjectives and see what happens.

Alisa: Well, for Marlene, I would say "dramatic."

Glen: Good, and for Little Bit?

Alisa: Sad, definitely sad.

Alisa identified the adjectives easily. After that, Glen had her add another dimension to the parts by labeling the adjectives as either positive or negative. At the end of the process, Alisa had developed the following parts, descriptions, and values.

Marlene Dietrich: dramatic (negative)
Little Bit: sad (negative)
Harriet: helpless (negative)
Eleanor Roosevelt: capable (positive)
Hillary Clinton: important (positive)
Lolita: funny (positive)

Partner: boring (negative)
Judge Judy: critical (negative)

Glen: I noticed you had a hard time deciding whether Lolita and Partner were positive or negative. Can you tell me more about the struggle you had?

Alisa: Well, Lolita may be funny and fun, but she also gets me into a lot of trouble. She is just not able to make commitments, and many of the relationships she sought out were not good for me.

Glen: Can you describe things about her that made you decide to call her positive?

Alisa: I guess it was the word *funny*. I mean, that is positive to me, and I did have a lot of fun. She has energy, and you know sex can be a lot of fun.

Glen: I can agree with that. So where does that put Partner?

Alisa: Well, the adjective is "boring," and boring is a real negative to me. But, at the same time, I really am happy as a partner, so I feel bad listing that part as totally negative.

Glen [*to the group*]: And that is important to remember. Even parts that we may see as negative often have positive meaning for us. Sometimes we are not aware of those positives, and sometimes we just do not allow ourselves see the part in that light.

[*To Alisa*]: Can you tell me the parts of Partner that you would describe as positive?

Alisa: I really like being in a committed relationship. Partner has all the security and support and caring that I think Lolita is always looking for but never could find. As Partner, I do miss the sex part, though.

Glen: Okay. Now, let's try one more part to see how a negative might also be a positive. Tell me about Judge Judy.

Alisa [*letting out a loud sigh*]: Well, she is a real large part of my life right now. I just hear her in my head going off with that loud, shrill voice, taking charge and telling all the other parts to shut up and listen to her.

Glen: Is she talking to you right now?

Alisa: Oh, yeah.

Glen: Can you tell me what she is saying?

Alisa [*in a loud, negative voice*]: This is really dumb. You keep making this up so you can be up here getting attention. There is nothing wrong with you, so just get on with your life and stop whining.

Glen: So, Judge Judy thinks you are okay?

Alisa: Well, I guess you could say that. I mean, every once in a while, she tells me how good things are, but that happened more when I was working. Judge Judy doesn't even deal with Little Bit, and Little Bit is around a lot right now.

Glen: And that is what we are here for today. By helping you know all your parts and understand their strengths and their weaknesses, you can begin to take charge of them. You can bring them together in a way that will help you succeed in this phase of your life.

So, can you tell me if there is anything about Judge Judy that you could see as positive?

Alisa: Well, when I was working, she really was a help. A lot of times, she kept me focused and kind of made me tougher and able to deal with the tough part of the job.

Glen: So she is the part of you that helps you focus and deal with tough things.

Alisa: Yeah, for a price, but yeah, she does that.

Glen [*looking at the chart*]: Right now, I see that we have a total of eight parts, and five of them you described as negatives.

Alisa: Yeah, that's a lot of negatives, isn't it?

Glen: Well, I think it reflects where you are right now and the struggle you are feeling. What we can do next is begin to work with the parts and use the Parts Party as a way to help you see each one, how they interact with each other, and then see if we can figure out how you can get them to work together. Do you feel like you are ready for that?

Alisa: I guess so.

Glen had completed the preparation phase of the Parts Party. The next phase involves setting up the party. Glen helped Alisa select people from the observers to represent each of the parts she had put on the list. Often, those who play these parts have known each other for many years and have a unique understanding of the individual doing the work as well as the techniques being used. The therapists also suggest words or actions that participants can use to increase their effectiveness.

Glen then asked this group to review the adjectives describing their respective parts. Several people asked questions to help clarify who and what they were representing. After answering the questions, Glen asked the group to get together at the side of the clearing, talk about their parts, and explore how they can work together to illustrate them and the way they relate or do not relate to each other part. While the group planned these aspects, Glen and Alisa stood together before the larger group of campers.

> Glen: Alisa, shall we make this your retirement party? It seems to me this occasion calls for a celebration. You have ended a successful career, and you are embarking on a new journey. Would you like your Parts to celebrate that reality?
>
> Alisa: Okay, yeah, that feels right to me. I did have a retirement party, but I was just there and kind of in shock and denial. I would like to really celebrate this time.
>
> Glen: Great, then let's do it. Where is the party happening?
>
> Alisa: I would like it outside in a park, kind of just like this, with lots of space and a big table full of wonderful food.
>
> Glen: Okay, let's make this area here the park and this row of chairs the party table. Now we will ask the guests to arrive and meet each other.
>
> [*To the parts*]: Are the guests ready?
>
> [*Those playing Alisa's parts discuss some last-minute details, and then turn and listens to Glen's instructions*]: You are all the guests at Alisa's retirement party. Some of you know each other a little, but most of you are strangers. I want you to come into this area just as if you are coming to a party and begin to introduce yourselves to the other parts at the party. Remember, you are attending Alisa's retirement party, so you may want to discuss that fact from the perspective of the part you represent.
>
> [*The parts walk to the front, and conversation and reactions swell up among them*].
>
> Judge Judy [*introducing herself to Hillary Clinton*]: My name is Judge Judy. I'm the person responsible for us making it this

far. I cannot believe we won't be working any more. We need that money. I just don't know how I am going to help out if she refuses to work.

Hillary Clinton: Well, I am H.C., and if you think you are responsible for our success, then you have no awareness of me and how hard I have worked. All that attention and success we had, just where do you think that came from? Who do you think made us read all those articles and keep calm when people kept calling us a bitch or said we were cold and heartless? I mean, it was all I could do to keep you all in check sometimes. I mean, what about the times we ended up going after some of those men at work?

Lolita [*joining them, and speaking to Hillary*]: I guess you must be talking about me again, you frigid over-achiever. A girl has got to have a little fun, and I really liked the last guy. Okay, so he was married . . . as far as I'm concerned, that's between him and the wife. I had nothing to do with that. Oh, Hillary, just back off and stop with that judgmental look.

Partner: Well, this seems like an interesting group. Hi, I'm Partner. I just arrived a few years ago. [*To Lolita, who is walking away*]. Okay, Lolita, go and disappear like you always do. We have finally found some happiness and contentment with a nice guy. If you can't deal with that, then take off. I'll just stay here and talk with these other women.

Judge Judy: I must say, you seem like a prim one, Partner, so smug and happy all the time. But I wonder when life in happy-ever-after land is going to get tiresome. Do you really think that wonderful man is going to keep wanting us when all you want to do is sit at home and eat bon bons?

Eleanor Roosevelt: Excuse me, I just heard that comment, Judge Judy, and I really wonder why you are so negative all the time? I think we just need to come together and make a competent woman. I mean, there is life for a woman after sixty. There are so many exciting things I can help us do. I can help us become a balanced, mature person. It is time that we all stop running around out of control or letting her [*indicating Hillary Clinton*] have all the control over us.

Hillary: Oh, give me a break. You think all I ever do is try to control things. Well, let me tell you, if I had not controlled things, do you really think we would have succeeded at anything? Without me, Lolita would have had us running around screwing our brains out.

Marlene [*striding into the group and interrupting with dramatic gestures and rapid, fervent speech*]: I say, have any of you noticed that old woman and little girl over there? The little girl looks like she is about to cry. She seems so shy, out of place, and almost frightened. And I just wonder why she keeps looking at that old woman. Well, I guess I know why. That woman is obviously senile and not even aware of what is going on. Sometimes I wonder if that's how we are all going to end up. If it is in the genes, there is nothing we can do about it, you know. I sure wish that child would just lighten up. Maybe if I go talk to her, I can help straighten her out.

Hillary [*sarcastically*]: Well, that should really help her. What she needs is some support and caring. . . . Remember, it takes a village.

Judge Judy: Oh god, Hillary, will you give it a rest? What she needs is a person to just make it clear to her that the child stuff is over and what comes next is not going to be pretty.

Eleanor: What I think she just needs is some recognition. I've never even met the child. Have any of you?

Judge Judy: Oh, god, yes. I spend all my time telling that little brat to shut up and go away.

Eleanor: Well, I have a unique idea. What if we all go and talk to the child and see why she is at this party anyway. I always have liked children, and Hillary, you communicate pretty well with kids. Shall we go meet her?

Hillary: Let's!

[*Hillary Clinton and Eleanor Roosevelt go over to Little Bit, who seems very shy in their presence*].

Eleanor: Hello, I'm Eleanor Roosevelt. What is your name, dear?

Little Bit [*very quietly, with her eyes on the ground*]: Uh, I'm Little Bit.

Eleanor: Do you get to come to these parties often?

Little Bit: Not really, I'm not even sure I'm allowed at this one.

Hillary: Well, for heaven's sake, why not? Oh, I'm sorry, honey, I'm Hillary Clinton, and I just want to be sure you are well taken care of.

Little Bit: Well, I don't like parties much. I only came 'cause I'm a part, I think.

Hillary: Well, how did you find out about the party?

Little Bit: From Harriet.

[*Eleanor and Hillary look at each other, startled*].

Eleanor: Well, I didn't think Harriet really knew. I mean, does she understand what is happening?

Little Bit: Oh, yeah, she and I talk to each other a lot. I know she's old, really old, but she knows more than you others realize. Some of the parts look down on her and laugh, and I don't think that's very nice. I know that Lolita and Partner don't like me at all, but Harriet, well, she—she's always nice to me when she has it together.

Hillary: Well, that's wonderful. But who else takes care of you? I don't remember meeting you before.

Little Bit: Most of the parts don't want to take care of a kid, so I don't come around too often. I kind of hang out with Harriet and see if I can get her to talk. Want to try and get her to talk to you?

Hillary [*after looking at Eleanor, who nods*]: Okay, why not? I always wonder about her.

[*The three move over to Harriet, who is slumped in a chair.*]

Eleanor: Oh dear, I think she is asleep. Maybe we shouldn't wake her.

Little Bit: It's okay. She always falls asleep when she is bored or left alone. Hey, Harriet, it's me, Little Bit, want to talk with me?

Harriet [*looking up slowly*]: Hello, Little Bit, this is a busy party isn't it? My, who are these parts?

Eleanor: I'm Eleanor Roosevelt, and this is Hillary Clinton.

Harriet: Oh, of course. I want to thank you for the great job you each did taking care of things during the time we were working. When I became a part, I felt so tired, and you just perked us all right up. And, Eleanor, I hope you will get stronger soon. See, my knees hurt so much right now that I can't let too much happen. And as the years go by, I think I will have to take over from you, probably more than you like.

Lolita [*joining the group*]: Hey, is that old lady really talking? I didn't think she could do anything! [*To Little Bit*]: Kid, what are you doing here? Haven't I told you to just go away so we can forget about you? You are always bringing things down around here. I mean, I even have to teach you how to play and stuff. What kind of a kid are you?

Glen intervened at this point to check in with Alisa and get her help giving directions to the parts. This also gave Alisa time to take in what she had been observing and hearing from the parts about their reactions. In the ensuing discussion, Glen helped refocus the issues and made sure that the party's direction and action made sense to Alisa.

Glen: FREEZE. Parts, please stay right where you are and exaggerate your physical stance so that it reflects how you are feeling. Now, Alisa, I want you to look at the whole scene and tell me what you see.

Alisa: It's interesting that Harriet and Little Bit are together with Eleanor and Hillary, and that Lolita is standing alone, almost opposite them. I would have thought Partner would have been more in the center of things. And I guess I would have Marlene more active, kind of in the center of the party.

Glen: Partner, please describe how you are feeling right now.

Partner: I feel very lonely without my partner. When he is not here, I feel empty and totally disconnected from the other parts, almost like I don't know how to be without him.

Alisa: Oh god, that is so right. Without Neal, that part is just a shell and not really present.

Glen: Okay. So, Partner, you continue to express those feelings and reflect them at the party. Marlene, let's hear how you are feeling.

Marlene: I'm not sure. I see all this connection over there, and I just don't know how it affects me.

Glen: Alisa, does what she said fit for you, or do you think she would have had a different reaction?

Alisa: The dramatic part of me is very threatened by Harriet and the way she is starting to take over my physical being. So, I think Marlene would try to stop those connections.

Glen: Okay, Marlene, I'd like you to join the conversation with Hillary, Eleanor, Little Bit, and Harriet and reflect the feelings Alisa just described.

[*Glen and Alisa step to the side and the party resumes*].

Marlene [*walking up to the group*]: Oh god, is Harriet awake? I mean, she and Little Bit just demand so much attention. I'm with you, Lolita, we need to get these two out of this party. Harriet, it is just too early for you to get this much attention. You are trying to take over, and it is *not* time for you. Little Bit, how many times have Lolita and I told you to stay away? Or, if you have to be with us, then be quiet? Oh god, don't start crying again. When are you going to grow up?

Judge Judy: Now look, all of you, this is getting a little out of hand. We cannot have all this conflict going on. Someone needs to be in charge or this is all going to spin out of control.

Glen [*noticing that Alisa is having an intense emotional reaction*]: FREEZE. Alisa, what is happening for you right now?

Alisa [*sobbing*]: Oh god, that is just how I feel. All the time, I feel out of control and that no one is in charge except maybe Harriet, and I do not *want* to be Harriet. . . . I can't be Harriet. [*More sobs*].

Glen: I think it could be good for you to actually see your parts go out of control. Maybe once you see what it looks like, we can work together to find a successful way for you to get control in a way that works better. Right now, it seems like you take control through denying a lot of these parts.

Alisa: I do feel like I'm always trying to control everything 'cause I'm so desperate that if I don't take control, everything will just spin away.

Glen: Do you think you could watch the parts spin out of control? [*She shakes her head*]. We don't have to, if you're not ready.

Well, here is another way we could try. First, we can get two people to come up here to be your support system. Then we can try having the parts start to go out of control and if you get overwhelmed, even with support, then you can stop the whole thing.

Alisa: Okay, I'll try that if you promise I can stop it if I need to.

Glen: I promise.

Two volunteers joined Alisa to provide her support, and Glen gave directions for the next part of the party.

Glen: Okay, let's continue with the conversation between Marlene, Judge Judy, Little Bit, Hillary, Eleanor, and Harriet. While you are talking, I'd like each of you to accentuate your viewpoint with your speech and your body. As they are talking, Partner, I would like you to spin around on the outside, and every now and then, see if you can get into the conversation. Finally, when the rest of you begin to feel things starting to come apart, I want you to spin out of the conversation but keep talking to yourselves.

Okay? Everyone ready? Alisa, you have your support in place? Let's begin.

Marlene, Judge Judy, Hillary, and Eleanor all spoke at once. Their voices increased in stridency and volume as Little Bit put her hands over her ears and hides behind Harriet. Partner circled the others, flapping her arms and weaving in and out of the group. The group ignored Partner's efforts and spoke louder.

Harriet [*over and over*]: Oh my goodness, oh my goodness. [*To the group*]: Now you hush, you just hush. Look how upset Little Bit is!

Judge Judy: This is *such* a waste of time. Why we ever came here is beyond me. There is no dealing with all these parts. Harriet is going to end up in charge, and I'm beginning to think the sooner, the better. [*She spins off*].

Marlene: Oh, what do you know, you stupid bitch judge. This life just sucks but it isn't 'cause we are getting old. Nobody listens anymore, and it seems like it's every part for itself. [*She turns her back but does not spin*].

Lolita: You know, if all of you would just listen to me, we could get out of here and have a little fun for a change. All of you are too damned scared of letting your feelings come out. So you know what, I'm out of here. [*She spins off in the opposite* direction, sometimes bumping into Judge Judy, who is spinning in one consistent direction].

Eleanor: Honestly, this is just too much bedlam. It is time to be mature and accept who you are. I can help us be an intelligent woman. I've already helped us live a good life up to now. I am ready for this new phase. Life is not that scary, and it does not have to be boring. There is so much to be done. I can help if these parts would just stop whining and get on with life. [*She holds her ground and does not spin*].

Hillary: I have really got to get out of here. This is too much chaos and bedlam. I mean, it could be fun to try to organize this, but who has the time or energy? I liked it a whole lot better when I just had control and could keep all the rest of these weirdo parts at bay. [*She goes to a spot away from all the others and spins in her own circle*].

Little Bit [*spinning into the center*]: Oh god, oh god, I knew this would happen. Now I'm going to be left here all alone. Everyone is yelling and having different ideas and going in different directions, and I cannot figure this out on my own. I'm so scared, I'm so scared!

Glen: FREEZE. Alisa, does any of this feel familiar?

Alisa [*her voice catching*]: Way too familiar.

Glen [*putting his arm around her reassuringly*]: Okay, and how are you feeling right now?

Alisa: Really identified with Little Bit. This is a repeat of what I felt a lot when I was little. However, I'm not as overwhelmed as I thought I would be. It really helps to see the chaos but to also see that even when everything is spinning, I have a center.

Glen: Where do you see the center?

Alisa: Well, for sure with Eleanor, who didn't leave; and I guess a little with Harriet, who is also still there and seems to be trying to relate to the rest of them.

During this discussion, the parts who moved outside the circle remained outside and Harriet, Eleanor, and Little Bit stood inside. Knowing that Alisa was feeling in control and agreed that what is being portrayed made sense, Glen moved into the next phase of the party.

Glen: I would like each of the parts to come to the front one at a time and share what it is you need or want from some or all of the other parts to help stop the bedlam or the spinning.

Hillary: I need everyone to listen to me so I can be the center and exert the control. I want to join with Eleanor and Partner and become better acquainted with Lolita and Little Bit.

Eleanor: I need everyone to be quiet, to speak one at a time, and to really listen to each other. I would like Hillary to join me in leading this group and supporting Little Bit and Partner and Lolita. I want Judge Judy to trust me and listen to me more.

Judge Judy: I need Hillary and Eleanor to take more responsibility so I don't have to be telling everyone what to do all the time. I want to be able to relax more and be a little more positive instead of always having to correct everything all the time.

Harriet: I want everyone to stop being so afraid of me and avoiding me. I want to be more awake and involved and feel less like some awful thing that everyone wants to avoid.

Partner: I want to be more than just a Partner. I need to exist on my own. I want support from Lolita to enjoy the sexual part of my life and to have more fun and be less needy.

Lolita: I want to have fun and feel less foolish and irresponsible. I want to bring joy into this phase of life. I want to join more with Partner and play with Little Bit . . . I think.

Little Bit: I want the other parts to see me and understand me. I want to be closer to Lolita and share in her fun. I want to help Partner play and be more childlike. I want the others to get to know Harriet.

Glen: Alisa, what do you see happening now? [*Involving Alisa at this point helps her discuss and then integrate what she has been observing*].

Alisa: I'm really surprised at how disconnected they all are. Yet, it also seems like they could become connected. It's like most of the parts hardly know each other. I'm also struck by how no one but Little Bit mentioned Harriet. I know that is my biggest struggle. Somehow, I have to integrate being an old woman, a really dependent old woman, into my life.

Glen: Would it be okay if we work on integrating that part?

Alisa [*very hesitantly*]: You mean have me get involved?

Glen: Yes, I think it's time for you to begin to interact with your parts and work with them to integrate Harriet into the group.

Alisa: I don't know. . . . That is so hard. Already I hear parts of me going "OH NO, I can't do that!'"

Glen: So . . . let's have the parts say that for you while you watch.

At this point, Alisa connected to what was happening but remained reluctant to take the next step in the process. Rather than push her, Glen decided to use the persons playing the parts to demonstrate what can happen. He was hopeful that as Alisa watched, she would relax and feel more comfortable about getting involved directly. Glen turned to the parts and asked them to talk about their ideas or feelings about integrating Harriet into their lives.

Marlene: I do not want to deal with this aging thing. I would rather die than get really old and helpless like that. I do not do helpless.

Judge Judy: I told you that was the outcome. Just face it. Besides, eventually you won't know what's going on anyway.

Eleanor: I don't know what the big deal is. I mean, everyone gets old, and that means you will become more dependent. But you can do things to make it better. You do things already. You exercise, and you work hard at staying involved, and who knows, maybe there will be a cure for Alzheimer's before you reach 85.

Hillary [*looking at Harriet*]: She doesn't look all that helpless to me. She seems more in touch than we may have realized.

Little Bit: I like Harriet a lot. She has lots more experience and information. I know she gets just as mad at all these other parts as I do. They just don't want to admit we exist.

Glen: FREEZE. Alisa, why don't we go and talk to Harriet and see what she has to say?

Alisa [*nods slowly, walks into the circle of parts, and faces Harriet, who is sitting in a chair*].

Harriet: Hello, Alisa, I have wanted to talk with you for a long time.

Alisa: I know I avoid you, and I'm sorry. I'm ready to listen to you now.

Harriet: I know you are scared of me because I am you and your future. I'm proud that you are trying so hard to make that future as positive as it can be for us. I know that our knees hurt and that it is my being elderly and having the arthritis that causes the pain and the fear for you. But you are doing things that will make it better and will make things less painful in the future.

Alisa: But I don't want to have to deal with pain!

Harriet: I know that, but I can't say it won't happen. What I know is that we are strong enough to deal with whatever will happen. I think every part of you can help us be happy and alive for every day that we have left.

Alisa: Can I hug you?

Harriet: You bet, and I promise you I will not break.

Glen then decided that it was time to sum up and end the work. In addition to the session's natural order, Glen also had to keep in mind the time and the fact that the people who had been observing the work had been sitting for several hours. Drawing Alisa to the middle of the circle, he addressed the parts who surrounded them.

Glen: At this time, we are going to help Alisa see how all of you are parts of her and can support her in this phase of her life. To do that, I would like all of you to make a sculpture of how you as a group can work together. Then Alisa and I will look at the sculpture you have created.

The parts move into groupings and then form a whole. Eleanor and Hillary quickly stand side by side, Lolita grabs Little Bit's hand, and Partner stands between Eleanor and Hillary, near Lolita and Little Bit. Harriet places herself on a chair in front of all of them. Judge Judy stands to the side of the group.

Glen: Alisa, what do you think of the sculpture?

Alisa: I like it. I like that Judge Judy is alongside the group rather than part of the group. I like that Partner is between all the others, and they are there to support her. [*She stops and cries but then continues*]. I also like that they are all in back of Harriet, and that they are there supporting her in her fragility. I think I have less fear of Harriet now that I know there is so much strength and love behind her.

Glen: Do you feel that you can accept all of these parts as part of you and who you are now as well as who you are becoming?

Alisa [*in a strong voice*]: Yes, and it really feels wonderful.

Glen: Then it is time to end the party. To do that, I would like each part to share a moment with you—not talking, but just being with you in silence. [*Each part stands with Alisa and then moves out of the circle until Alisa and Glen stand alone.*]

At the end of each work session that involves volunteers from the group, the therapist takes time to "de-role" each volunteer. Generally, this is done with the following phrases.

> Please give yourself an appreciation for helping [Alisa] by taking on this role. Now, I would like you to symbolically take off the mantle of the role that you assumed and, together, say your name. You are no longer in that role and can now return to your own self and your place here at camp.

Generally, those persons who have played the roles also briefly discuss how the role affected them and what lessons they learned for themselves while playing the role. Following the discussion by the role players, the facilitator allows time for group feedback.

Glen [*to the group at large*]: I am going to have Alisa sit with me and give each of you a chance to respond to the work. Let me remind you of the guideline for your response. This is your opportunity to talk about how the work has affected you and to discuss anything that has bubbled up for you. Alisa has taken in a great deal in the last few hours. Rather than add to that input, we want Alisa to have time to absorb what happened and give this time to each of you to process whatever came up for you.

Carl: This work had great meaning for me. I realize that I have struggled with finding the strength to start a new phase of my life. I'm tired, and I know I'm done with work, but I also have a Harriet in my life called Harold. My father has Alzheimer's, and I'm so afraid that Harold is out there waiting for me. Watching this work has helped me realize that I have many parts to support me as I am aging. Thank you for helping me see that more clearly.

Cynthia: This work was so powerful for me. I'm trying to support my mother, who has just retired and is struggling with depression. Sometimes when she says she wishes she had never retired, I get so frustrated with her. I thought she would just get involved in activities and be as busy as she was when she worked. Instead, she seems unable to do anything. This work helped me see how conflicted she must be, and I think I can be more supportive now that I have that understanding.

Vince: This is the first Parts Party I've watched at camp. I was struck by how powerful the tool is. I know that we all have different parts, but this work really made clear what that means and how conflicted those parts can become. I have a lot of thinking to do about the parts in me and how I can work at getting them better integrated.

Rich: This work helped me understand the conflicts I have inside of me. Thank you.

Glen [*after everyone had spoken*]: I would like all of you to close your eyes and think of the many parts that we have within us. As you see and feel these parts, give yourself permission to take from this work ideas and thoughts and experiences that can help you become more aware of the parts and accept them. [*He pauses for a short silence*].

Also, become aware of the energy from the earth and from the heavens, and breathe in the quiet of this wonderful place. When you are ready, slowly open your eyes and let us all join the larger world and its many parts.

People who experience the Parts Party consider this technique one of Virginia's most powerful tools. By observing the different parts interact, a person has the opportunity to become aware of the parts and how they affect other parts. He or she also becomes freer to make choices about how to use those parts.

When people do this type of work at camp, members of the community forge deep connections. These connections then lead to even more powerful work. As one long-time camper disclosed:

> I am always amazed at the power of the work we do at camp. Originally, it seemed to be Virginia's magic, but as we have matured as a community, I think it has more to do with how well we know each other and how committed we are to participate in the work and make it real for the person. Many of us have become very effective in knowing how to do techniques like Parts Party and Family Reconstruction. Of course, the therapists are still the key ingredient, but our living and working together makes the work much stronger.

Another camper remarked:

> It's just so striking how people participate in the work and just seem to say the right thing at the right moment. That is particularly true with the Parts Party. When things don't come together, it's usually because the person doing the work is new and we just don't know them well enough to help bring out the right thing . . . . That's when the therapists' skills become really important. They need to know when to stop the work and get it back on track. A lot of times they will stop and ask the person doing the work to help tell the parts what to do or tell them what to say. But when we know each other well, we can really become that part, and then the work is just magical.

Glen, the therapist, said:

> Doing a Parts Party at camp is challenging. We do not have the time to prepare as much as we would in, say, a Process Community. Work is always more powerful when we know the person doing the work, and at camp, we get to know each other pretty well. But the technique itself is powerful enough that we can also just trust the process to unfold. I always check in with the person doing the work and make sure that what is happening feels right to them, and when it does not, then I have the person tell me what needs to change.
>
> When you work with Virginia's techniques, you really have to stay with the process and respond intuitively. It does not always go as we hope, but I am amazed how often things just unfold before us.

Family Reconstruction

Family Reconstruction is a therapeutic tool that Virginia created to help people become aware of childhood events that they could not understand when they were children. By helping the participant learn about the puzzles of his or her early life, Family Reconstruction frees the participant from behavior that may be limiting his or her ability to function as an adult. Family Reconstruction can also correct early childhood experiences. Children who were rejected, abused, or attacked emotionally get to experience positive nurturing and learn how, as adults, to continue providing that nurturance to the injured child who is still a part of them.

A complete Family Reconstruction involves a number of steps that are designed to elicit information about the participant (called the "Star"), his or her family and Circle of Influence (significant persons in the Star's life). Like the Parts Party, this technique must be adapted to a much briefer time when used at SFC. During a work session there, therapists may use part of the Family Reconstruction process as one of several techniques, or it may be the only technique in the entire session. The following story illustrates how Family Reconstruction can be adapted for use at SFC. This story is based on work done at camp. It is not a recreation of any particular work or events.

Stefan's Story

Stefan, age 26, asked to do a work session to deal with anger he had been struggling with throughout his life, particularly in close relationships. Stefan asked Nita to be the primary therapist for the work and also requested that Lincoln participate as well. As the work session began, Nita and Stefan stood at the front of the amphitheater.

> Nita: Stefan, can you describe the problem you want to work on today?
>
> Stefan: Well, last year I remember watching someone work—I think it was Nelson—about anger, and I realized that is something I really struggle with. Watching Nelson let go of his anger gave me such a release that I knew I needed to do some work.
>
> Nita: So you want to create an opportunity to express the anger you feel?

Stefan: Well, that's part of it, but I also want to look at what is causing the anger as well, and I guess put the anger where it belongs instead of just having it come out all over everywhere.

Nita: And do you have ideas about whom or what you are angry about?

Stefan [*slowly but with strong feeling*]: Yeah, I know . . . I'm mad at my dad.

Nita [*quietly*]: And do you know why you are angry at your dad?

Stefan [*with quiet fury*]: I'd have to say because he molested me . . . a lot when I was young.

Nita: Yes, I'd say that is something to be angry about.

Stefan [*in the same tone*]: You bet, real angry.

Nita: Can you tell us where in your body that you feel the anger?

Stefan: I guess mostly in my gut, and in my jaw.

Nita: I notice you have your hands are clenched and you seem to be breathing real hard

Stefan: Yeah, I just feel like I want to beat the shit out of something.

Nita: Well, we want to help you work with that anger today. You asked for both Lincoln and me to work with you, so I'm going to have Lincoln join us now. Is that okay with you?

Stefan: Sure.

Nita [*after conferring briefly with Lincoln*]: Stefan, we would like you to remember a time when you were with your father and you got really angry. Do you think you can do that?

Stefan [*after thinking awhile and then nodding*]: Okay, I remember one time when I was really young.

Nita: All right. Now, can you describe the memory?

Stefan: You mean what happened?

Nita: Well, let's start with who is in the memory.

Stefan: Just my dad and me.

Nita: Okay, and how old are you?

Stefan: I think about six.

Nita: And your dad would have been————?

Stefan: Maybe twenty-eight or twenty-nine.

Nita: Good. So, what we will do next is create a scene of that memory, and to do that, we need you to pick someone to be you as a little boy and then someone to be your father.

Stefan: I don't know, I just don't think I can ask anyone to do that. I mean, this isn't a very good memory.

Nita: Well, let's see if there are people in the audience who will be willing to be your little boy, even knowing that your memory is painful, and then you pick from that group and trust that whomever you pick will take care of him- or herself.

Stefan: That feels better to me.

Nita [*to the group*]: Will anyone who is willing to be Little Stefan and feels that they can protect themselves while playing this role please raise your hand? [*Many people raise their hands*].

Okay, please keep your hands up. Stefan, I would like you to pick someone from the group that has their hands raised.

Stefan looks around the group, smiling as he sees how many people have raised their hands. He decides upon Sean, a young adult who is slender and looks quite young. Sean comes forward.

Stefan: Are you sure, Sean? I mean, I don't want to make this hard on you. [*Sean assures Stefan*].

Nita: Stefan, are you able to accept Sean's reassurance? This is important. This is your work, and I want you to put all of your energy into experiencing the work without having to worry about someone else.

Stefan: I know I do that a lot. I feel so intensely that I forget that other people experience things their own way. It's like this feeling I have just takes over the whole world.

Nita: Yes, these kinds of feelings are body feelings, and they come from a very early experience when your basic survival is threatened, which makes them so powerful. Virginia created ways to help you recreate the original experience so that you can observe the experience as an adult rather than a child. As an adult, you are more equipped to understand what happened to you and to help that child who is still a part of you. Our goal is to have you understand how your anger began so that when you encounter these feelings in your adult life, you can make decisions as to whether the anger is from the present or from your past.

Stefan: Yeah, I get that.

Nita: Good, and now can you pick out someone to be your father?

Stefan: Oh, I don't. . . . Okay, but will you ask for volunteers again, this time for my father?

Nita does as he asks. Men in the group volunteer, and Stefan picks Paul. Paul expresses his willingness to assume the role, and Stefan agrees to accept assurances that Paul will protect himself.

Nita: Okay [*pointing to the two volunteers*], so here are Little Stefan and his dad. Now, I want Lincoln to be with you, Stefan. He is here to help be my guide as we set up a scene to show what happen between Little Stefan and your father.

Stefan [*very hesitantly*]: Well, the memory is about when he molested me.

Nita [*gently*]: Okay, and can you tell me the first time you remember your father doing that?

Stefan [*speaking with difficulty*]: I guess I was about 6 years old.

Nita: And where were you?

Stefan [*sounding confused*]: Where was I?

Nita: In this memory, are you in some particular place?

Stefan [*after thinking a moment*]: Yeah, I was in my bedroom.

Nita: Stefan, what is happening right now? You just clenched your fists, and your whole body looks very tense.

Stefan [*visibly trying to maintain control, shaking, and almost in a growl*]: No, no, no.

Lincoln [*putting an arm around Stefan*]: Stefan, I'm here with you. Together, we are going to remember little Stefan, the boy, but we are here on the outside looking in, not back in your bedroom.

Stefan [*letting out a big sigh*]: Thank you. I need to remember that, I just know I cannot go back there. I am here with you, not in that bedroom.

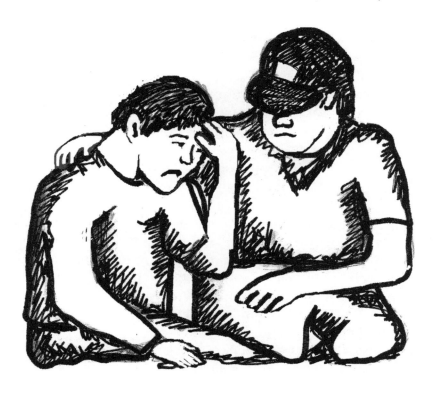

Lincoln: That's right. Now, is there some kind of signal we can use that will let me know when you feel like you are slipping from here with me into the bedroom?

Stefan: How about we hold hands and when it starts to happen, I can squeeze your hand?

Lincoln: That sounds fine. And when you squeeze my hand, I want you to remind yourself that you are here with me, and I will help you stay here and make sure you are protected.

Stefan: Okay, that feels much better. I think I can do this if I don't go back into that room. [*He begins to shake*].

Lincoln [*pulling him close*]: Okay, now squeeze my hand. [*Stefan does. Lincoln leans over and whispers into Stefan's ear*]: You are here with me, and I will make sure you are safe.

Stefan: Okay.

Nita [*in a comforting tone*]: Now, we know that Little Stefan is around six years old, and he is in the bedroom. So we will make this space over here the bedroom. Can you tell me what is in the bedroom?

Stefan [*pointing to the designated space*]: There is a bed against the wall.

Nita: Okay, is there more furniture in the bedroom?

Stefan: There's a desk and a dresser against the opposite wall.

Nita: Okay, and where is the door? [*Turning from setting the scene, she sees that Stefan looks upset and agitated*]. Stefan, what is happening with your body right now?

Stefan: I just feel so tight and like I can't breathe. I think I'm going to pass out.

Lincoln: Let's sit down over here. Okay, now breathe in and out very slowly. Okay, in and out. Is that feeling better?

Stefan [*catching his breath and speaking in a more normal tone*]: Yeah, I think I'll be okay if I can sit instead of stand.

Nita: That's fine. Are you sure you're ready to continue? [*Stefan nods*]. I think we were deciding where the door is to the room.

Stefan: It's across from the bed.

Nita [*after drawing a line to signify the doorway and an X for the dresser and desk*]: Now, Stefan, can you look at the space and visualize your bedroom? [*Stefan nods, tenses up again, and squeezes Lincoln's hand. Lincoln leans over and whispers in his ear, and Stefan nods*].

Stefan: Okay, I can see it . . . not sure I want to, but I can see it.

Nita [*softly, with great gentleness*]: Stefan, can you tell us the story of what happens in the bedroom?

Stefan: Well, I was in my bed; it must have been nighttime. I remember I had this awful stomach ache. . . . Oh god [*he leans over and retches*].

Lincoln comes around quickly and holds Stefan encouraging him to take deep breaths. Lincoln holds Stefan, quietly telling him that everything is okay and that he will take care of him.

Nita instructs Little Stefan, who is lying on the ground in the area designated as the bed, to hold on to his stomach and moan quietly.

Nita [*after Stefan calms*]: Stefan, I would like you to look at the bedroom again and let me know if this looks like your memory.

[*Stefan nods but then shakes his head*].

Nita: No? Okay, what needs to be different?

Stefan: I would never have moaned or made a sound. It's good that he's holding his stomach, but I would never have moaned. If my father heard any kind of sissy sound, he would have been on me in a minute.

Nita instructs Little Stefan to hold his belly in silence. Without a sound, Little Stefan makes very clear the pain he is feeling.

Nita: So this little boy who has a stomachache has to be very quiet to make sure that no one will know that he is hurting?

Stefan [*with great bitterness*]: Yeah, that's about right. And I had a lot of stomachaches. Just about every night I went to bed, my stomach hurt.

Nita: Do you remember why? Did you have some type of physical problem?

Stefan: No, I don't think so. I think it was just so tense whenever we ate dinner or were together anywhere as a family. My mother and I . . . we were always waiting for my father to blow up and start screaming and then hitting. So by the end of the meal, I always had a stomachache.

Nita: Well, that's not surprising. With that kind of environment at mealtime, it would certainly be difficult for a little boy not to get tense and feel pain in his belly. Can you tell us what else Little Stefan is feeling? Anything else besides a pain in his belly?

Stefan: I guess he's wondering if his mother or his father is going to come in to say good night.

Nita: Who does he want to come in to say good night?

Stefan [*in a young, panicked voice*]: I want mommy. Please don't let it be daddy. [*He squeezes Lincoln's hand again and then doubles over, holding his gut. After Lincoln helps him catch his breath, he looks up and nods to Nita that he is ready to begin again*].

Nita: So we have Little Stefan on his bed, holding his belly and hoping his mother will come in to say good night but very afraid that his daddy will come instead of his mother. It sounds to me that Little Stefan not only hurts but he feels very afraid. Does that fit, Stefan, that there is a really strong feeling of fear, of your father?

Stefan [*covering his eyes*]: Oh yes, he is so scared cause he knows his mommy won't come. That *he* won't let her come that only *he* gets to tell him goodnight. . . . Oh, it hurts, it hurts. [*Lincoln holds Stefan, who is moaning*].

Nita [*after conferring with Eliana*]: Are there some men in the group willing to come up and stand behind Lincoln and Stefan to provide him with more support? [*Almost every man volunteers, and Nita suggests that four join them*].

Stefan, these men are members of your Satir Family Camp family. They are here to to make sure that you are safe. Where would you like them to be so that they can give you more safety?

Stefan [*resuming more control*]: Yeah, that's good. I guess I want them to stand all around us.

Nita: Okay, let's have some on each side and some in the back Does that feel right?

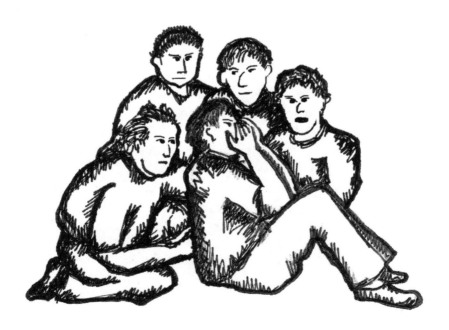

Stefan: Yeah, that's much better.

The four men [*leaning over and speaking together, as Eliana has instructed them to say*]: We will keep you safe. We will keep you with us. You are with us. We will not let him hurt you. [*Stefan leans back into Lincoln and looks at the faces of the men*].

Nita: Stefan, are you able to take in the support and safety that these men give you?

Stefan [*breathing deeply and smiling*]: Yes, that makes it much better!

Nita [*gently*]: Do you feel that you are ready to tell us what happens next in the bedroom?

Stefan [*with hands over his face, in a racing voice*]: My father comes in and says I better not be whining 'cause he hates me whining. So I roll over and try to let go of my belly, but I start crying and then he pulls at me and forces me on my stomach and says it's time I learn what it means to be a little sissy, and then he climbs on top of me and I can't breathe 'cause he's so heavy and———

Stefan [*rising to a shriek*]: Oh god, it hurts, it hurts, it hurts!

Stefan falls out of the chair onto the ground, lying in a fetal position on his side with his arms locked around his knees, sobbing uncontrollably. Both therapists sit down next to him and encourage him to let out the feelings.

Lincoln: Yes, it hurts, and it is okay for you to express that hurt. It's okay for you to cry and scream.

The four men [*after Nita motions them to sit around Stefan*]: It's okay for little boys to cry. It is okay for little boys to be sad and scared. Little boys need to be cared for and cherished. Little boys need fathers who do not use them. Little boys need fathers who love and protect them. If we had been with you, we would have protected you. We would not have let him hurt you like that.

Stefan [*after regaining control, sitting up, and looking around at the faces surrounding him*]: It is so hard to remember that. Why weren't you there when it happened? [*He leans over and sobs again*].

Nita: You are so right, Stefan. This abuse is so difficult for a child to endure. You were scared and hurt, and one of the people you depended on for your survival is the person that is hurting you. It was not fair, and you had every right to be hurt and scared.

But when you feel ready, I would like you to look at all the men who are surrounding you now and offering you all the positive caring and love that they have to give you. When you can, I want you to take in that love and support so that we can help you help this little boy who is still in the bedroom with your father.

Stefan [*after taking some time to absorb the sight and sense of the men around him, and rising to sit in a chair again*]: It is just so wonderful to look at all these male faces and feel goodness instead of evil. I just see acceptance and caring. I don't think I have ever felt safe with a man before.

Nita: There are many men who are here for you, not only during this work but also during the week here at camp and throughout the year. There are many good men who are able to give you this support whenever you need it.

Stefan [*after spending more time taking in the faces of the men around him and then sitting back with a large sigh and a big smile*]: Well, that was great. . . . So I'm cured, right?

Nita [*laughing*]: Well, that was a huge beginning, but I'm thinking we need to take another step that I hope will help you begin to take care your little boy.

Stefan: I'm not sure I like where this is going.

Nita: Then let's slow down and make sure you are comfortable. I don't want to do anything that you feel you are not ready for or choose to do.

Stefan: I guess I know there's another part of this, especially if I'm going to do anything about the anger.

Nita: And what do you know?

Stefan: That I need to deal with my father. [*He again clenches his fists*].

Nita: Stefan, can you tell me what you are feeling in your body right now?

Stefan [*through clenched teeth*]: I just feel so angry. [*He pours out his words*]: All those years, he just used me over and over.

You know, I did try to confront him just before he died. I had not talked to him since I left home when I was eighteen, but when I heard he was dying, I went to see him in the hospital. When I got there, I found this wizened old man lying in a bed hooked up to all these machines. It was so ironic just when I finally decided to tell the son of a bitch what I thought of him, *he* is so out of it I don't think he even knew I was there.

It took all my courage to just go in and look at him. I think I said something like "I hope you rot in hell," and then I walked out. And when I got to the car, I put my fist through the side window. Cost me some bucks to fix it and didn't give me one bit of relief.

Nita: So maybe there is something we can do here that will bring you some relief.

Stefan: What are you thinking about?

Nita: We can begin this next part of the work by having your father go into the bedroom and be with Little Stefan.

Stefan [*moving away rapidly*]: Oh god, I guess so. I just start to feel so little when that happens.

Nita: That makes sense. Many of your feelings are very vulnerable, but I wonder if Little Stefan didn't get angry as well?

Stefan: I don't remember that. . . . I just remember being scared and hurt and . . . oh god, I hurt!!

Lincoln [*coming up to Stefan and motioning the four men closer*]: Stefan, hold my hand and squeeze. Remember you are *not* in the bedroom. You are with me and with your support group, and we are going to make sure that no one hurts you.

Stefan: Okay, I remember. [*He looks around at the group of men, who smile back at him*]. Okay, I have your support. Okay, I can do this. [*To Nita*]: Uh, what is that we are doing now?

Nita [*gently*]: I would like you to help me set up the scene in the bedroom with both Little Stefan and your father.

Stefan: You mean when he molests me?

Nita: If that is what you remember. What we want to do is give you a chance to look at this scene and then we want to help you tell your father what you think about what happened and how you feel about it.

Stefan: Oh man . . . it is so hard to see it.

Nita [*quietly and kindly*]: Yes, it is, but this scene has always been with you, Stefan, and this time we want you to see it not as the little boy but as the man you are today and with the support that you have here in this community.

Stefan [*taking a deep breath*]: I guess, then, we have to have Little Stefan lying down against the wall. He would have his face to the wall. [*Little Stefan takes his position*]. Yeah, and he is kind of pulled up in a ball. His knees are against his chest. I remember I used to hope that I could just disappear. [*He cries, and Lincoln squeezes his hand and motions the men to speak*].

The four men: It's okay for little boys to cry. It's okay for little boys to be sad and scared. Little boys need to be cared for and cherished. Little boys need fathers that do not use them. Little boys need fathers who love and protect them. If we had been with you, we would have protected you. We would not have let him hurt you like that.

Nita [*as Stefan controls his tears*]: Can you describe what your father does next?

Stefan: He . . . he comes in the room and he's yelling.

Nita: What is he yelling?

Stefan [*loudly*]: You sniffling little sissy. You—you—just be quiet! You are always complaining, and I have to come up here and deal with you. Why can't you be a man?

The father [*picking up the taunts*]: You are such a sissy, You don't know how to be a man. I'll teach you to be so whiny. I'll show you what happens to sissies.

Stefan [*putting his hands over his ears and sobbing*]: Oh god, that is him. That is exactly like him. It is so scary! He is going to grab me. . . . Oh god.

[*Nita instructs the father to pull at Little Stefan*].

Stefan [*in a strangled voice, hiding his head in Lincoln's shoulder*]: I can't watch. I can't watch.

Lincoln: You don't need to. We will watch and protect you and help you. And when you are ready, we will be there to help you confront him.

[*The father looms over Little Stefan, pulls on his shoulder, and tries to lift him. Eliana confers with Little Stefan*].

Little Stefan [*shouting*]: No! Leave me alone, leave me alone. Don't hurt me. Don't hurt me!

Stefan [*first shrinking from the sounds and sights and then, after several repetitions by Little Stefan*]: You know, I suddenly remember I did yell. I did try to stop him. I always thought I was such a coward and a sissy because he always called me that, but I was not. I did try to stop him.

Nita: Do you think you can come and stand with me now and look at the scene?

Stefan [*motioning toward the four men*]: Can I bring them with me?

Nita: Absolutely.

[*The group comes and stands by Nita and looks at the scene of the boy resisting the father*].

Little Stefan [*yelling*]: No! *No!*

Father [*yelling*]: You sniffling little sissy. Just be quiet. You are always complaining, and I have to come up here and deal with you. Why can't you be a man?

Stefan [*in a stronger and angry voice*]: Yeah, you were such a man. All you could do was fuck little boys to show what a man you were. [*He shouts more and more loudly*]: You were a horrible father. I hated you. I wanted you to die. Every time you touched me, I wanted to kill you. I wish I had killed you instead of the cancer. You should have suffered for years instead of just a few months.

The four men [*taking up the words, at Lincoln's instruction*]: I hate you. You hurt me. You had no right to do those things to me. You were not a father, a father does not hurt his son. You were wrong. It was not my fault. I needed someone to love me, not fuck me.

Stefan [*sobbing as he becomes aware of what the men are saying, he falls to the ground. His sobs grow from tears to screams of rage. Lincoln and the other men surround him. As Lincoln holds Stefan, all the men encourage Stefan to release the rage. Stefan hits a pillow placed in front of him. After a few smacks, he stops and says*]: I need something stronger. I want a stick, a big stick that I can use to just club him. I want to club him out of my life.

[*Stefan hits the pillow with a walking stick provided by a camper. He shouts*]: You tried to ruin my life! I am not like you, I love my son and I won't let anyone hurt him.

Lincoln [*supplying more words*]: You had the problem, not me. You should have cared for me. You put your needs first and used me.

Stefan [*bursting into uncontrollable yells*]: I hate you, I hate you, I hate you! [*Spent, he falls on his knees over the pillow, which is pretty well demolished. As he calms, he looks up and jokes*]: Sorry about the pillow. [*Laughter*].

Nita [*after assuring Stefan that the pillow can be replaced, and helping Stefan up*]: Stefan, can we have your father leave the room so you can talk with Little Stefan?

Stefan [*with relief in his voice*]: Yes, please get him out of there.

[*The father leaves, Little Stefan sits up, and Stefan sits in a chair facing him*].

Nita: Little Stefan, are there things you want to tell Stefan?

Little Stefan: I was really glad to see you get so angry about what happened. I know you get angry a lot, but it is never because of the real thing. It's like what happened to me just doesn't exist for you.

Stefan: You are right about that. I just wanted to forget and pretend as if it never happened. As soon as I got out of that house, I decided it just never happened.

Little Stefan: But I'm still here. I am here locked up in your anger. Even if you do not remember it, I feel like every time you get angry, it happens again for me. I feel so trapped. I want to be free, too!

Stefan: But I feel like if I remember, then I go back there. . . . [*He covers his face with his hands*].

Nita [*very gently*]: And then what?

Stefan [*in great sobs*]: Then I will be what he said. A big sissy, just a big queer.

Nita: You know, Stefan, many boys who have been molested feel that means they are homosexuals. Some may be, and others may not be. What your father did to you does not define who you are. It does not define your sexuality, and it does not define your personality.

Stefan: I know that. I know I believe that . . . but I just never have been able to feel that.

Nita: And until you are able to reconnect with this little boy, you probably won't be able to feel that.

Stefan [*reaching out, taking little Stefan's hands, and speaking to him in a very tender voice*]: Little Stefan, I know you are a little boy who survived horrible abuse. I want to be able to see you as I see Nicky [Stefan's son], just a little boy doing what little boys do. All that other stuff *he* put into my head. That was *his* stuff, *his* problems. I can let it go and just be with you, a wonderful innocent little boy.

Nita [*to the group as a whole*]: Virginia knew that our inner child must continue to seek care and support, particularly when we did not get the care and love we both needed and deserved as a child. As adults, we need to provide ourselves with that love and care before we fully enter into an intimate relationship with another adult. Like Stefan, we are often raging, hurting, or struggling over things in the present that really belong to the past.

Stefan, this work has allowed you to relive your experiences as a child and to express the rage that you felt—both as a child and as a man—because of those experiences. You have made a wonderful beginning in reconnecting to your child. You have taken the first step in caring for Little Stefan as well as the first step on your journey toward health.

Stefan: I know this is just the beginning, but I feel like this huge burden has been lifted from me.

Nita [*giving him a big hug*]: That's wonderful. Are you okay if we stop here and have people who have been watching talk about how this work has affected them?

Stefan: Okay. [*He sits beside Lincoln*].

[Sean and Paul provide feedback about their experience in the roles of Little Stefan and Stefan's father. The four men who provided support also comment].

Nita [*to the larger group*]: This is a time for each of you to talk about how this work has affected you. Please focus your remarks on how you responded. You may want to give feedback about Stefan, but this is a time for Stefan to stay with his own feelings and for those of you who have been affected to talk about your feelings.

Therapist Response

To understand Virginia's methods and the way they are used at camp, it helps to get the perspective of a therapist regarding that work. The following is a discussion by Nita regarding Stefan's work.

> Whenever we do a work session about molestation, I am challenged by the pain and emotion that is generated—not just for the person doing the work but for everyone who participates in the work itself as well as those watching. Virginia's methods help people re-experience childhood emotions in ways that are often overwhelming. I think camp is such a valuable place to work on these issues because of the safety it provides both during the work and afterward.
>
> I think it is important that we, the therapists, know the person doing the work. When we have time to be with a person at camp, both in formal sessions and in the many informal times that occur during the week, we get to know the person in ways that help us make the work more personal and therefore more successful. Much of the work we do here is intuitive. Virginia's techniques are our primary tools, but those tools are more valuable when we can use our knowledge of the person as well. You just intuitively know what approach will work and what words will have the most meaning.
>
> For example, to give Stefan support, Lincoln uses particular phrases. He is able to have the men use other phrases that he knows will have meaning to Stefan. It's not like Stefan had told Lincoln exactly what had gone on with his father. Rather Stefan and Lincoln have spent time together in men's group and playing ping-pong and just hanging out, so Lincoln has a very real sense of who Stefan is. The same is true for Sean. He and Stefan have become good friends at camp. In fact, Stefan first shared what happened to him with Sean. Sean was the first person to help Stefan begin to deal with the aftermath of that abuse. I also worked with Stefan on an individual basis over the past two camps before he decided to work at camp. We all had this rich understanding of Stefan before we began the work that he did at camp this summer.
>
> Doing this kind of work at camp offers a therapist so many unique ways to help people. We have a large group of people to choose among for role players, and they bring their understanding and awareness of both the person who is doing the work as well as their knowledge about how work is done at camp. It's kind of a joke among camp that when a dad is needed, Paul gets chosen. And he

really is an ideal person. He has the gray hair, beard, and mustache and can take on a personality so well. Sometimes Paul is a caring giving dad, but he is also good at being remote and distant; and in this work, he was truly scary as an abusive father. It is sometimes uncanny how people select someone who is perfect for the role. That is the strength of Virginia's technique, of course, but it seems to be even more powerful here. People come here year after year and become very skilled at using these techniques, particularly role playing.

There can also be risks doing such intense work, particularly when it involves child molestation. Some people are not ready or just cannot take on certain roles. In this work, Stefan had difficulty asking people to participate, so we took the time to make sure that he understood that people who volunteer to assist in the work can and will protect themselves.

Therapists also have to watch for the effect of this kind of work on observers as well as participants. Many adults who were molested as children survive by pushing the experience out of their conscious memory. Then they may watch someone and their own memories may get triggered. Fortunately, if that happens, we can help that person as well. We have a large team of therapists as well as skilled members in the community who are available to help people deal with things that come up during the week. We always leave time at the end of a work session to allow people to talk about how the work has affected them. When we notice someone has been affected by the work, we check in with them individually to be sure they are okay.

Working with a team of therapists is important to me. I know Virginia was a remarkable therapist, but I have trouble imagining how she did this work all by herself. For the rest of us mere mortals, the team is critical for our own survival. First, there are all the groups we try to meet with: the children, the teens, the young adults and men and women's groups. But more important than having the bodies to go around is having different therapists, men and women, who come with different experiences and viewpoints but who can also work together to provide the best and richest experience to the camp. Each therapist contributes his or her thoughts and responses during sessions.

In this work, Eliana was not leading the work, but she was present throughout and on several occasions was able to provide words or ideas that neither Lincoln nor I could have contributed because we were so actively involved. We are sensitive not to interfere with each other, but we are also comfortable and able to ask or offer each other ideas whenever that is needed or will add to the situation.

Virginia taught therapists that the person doing the work, not the therapist, is in charge of what happens during the work. She knew that if anything meaningful is going to happen during a session, the person doing the work has to decide what that will be. It is very easy to get caught up in the emotion and the drama of this kind of work. That makes it incumbent on the therapist to check in with the person doing the work and make sure we are not getting ahead of them. Sometimes people decide not to go further in a session even when it seems obvious to us, the therapists, that they need to take the next step to make meaningful change.

I had originally thought this work would be a more traditional Family Reconstruction and we would help Stefan understand his parents, particularly his mother. But we never even addressed where his mother was during that part of his life. Some of the problem was that time was limited, but he never raised her, and I had an intuitive sense that at least for this work the mother's role was not significant. I am sure Stefan will do work again on this issue, and it is likely he will be ready to address his mother. We can also do more about why his parents parented the way they did.

To be honest, it was tempting for me as the therapist to raise his mother because I know that the non-offending parent often has an impact on the child that is as significant as, if not more than, the abuser. I could have treated Stefan's not mentioning her as avoidance and pushed the issue. But in the end, that would have been meeting my need rather than Stefan's. When you use Virginia's methods, the person doing the work is in charge of the direction, not the therapist.

Satir treatment modalities are the force that unifies the SFC community. The strong connections and bonds within the community come from the therapeutic work that is done at every level of interaction. From the time spent talking and performing tasks together to the time spent working on therapeutic issues, SFC grows and develops out of the wisdom of Virginia Satir. The concepts and theory inherent in each application provide a greater understanding of the belief she had in a human's ability to grow and overcome any trauma or deficit.

10

Taking Satir Family Camp into the World

Virginia eventually expanded the focus of her work from families to communities to countries. As one camper relates:

> Virginia believed that communities—be they local, state, or national—form at the family unit. She also believed that these communities could foster fully human beings in the same way that an individual family fosters the growth of its members. She chose to focus much of her international work on Russia and the countries that were part of the Soviet Union because she saw the chaos and breakdown during the shift in those countries' governments and societies. Virginia believed that she could heal these societies by helping them to rebuild the family unit.

In the same way, sfc participants take the knowledge and skills they learn at sfc into their lives outside camp. At a 2005 Free University session, campers shared how they apply sfc principles and methods in their daily lives. The following stories illustrate how Virginia's experiment continues to be carried out into the world. The first is from a long-time camper and pediatrician:

> The first Satir technique I used at work was Temperature Reading. When I became chief of pediatric services, we operated in a typical hierarchical structure with the doctors in charge. At that time, the office staff didn't attend the weekly staff meetings. I expected everyone to attend the staff meeting and encouraged the office staff to participate as full equals to the doctors. I began the meeting by having people share Appreciations. It's amazing how just that one

thing can change the atmosphere of a meeting and eventually the organization. At first, the Appreciations were awkward and kind of artificial, but as they got used to it, people began to notice positive things and actually save them up for sharing at the staff meeting. After Appreciations worked, I added time for Puzzles and Bugs, Hopes and Wishes and, of course, New Information. The more we used this technique, the more change I saw, particularly in the office staff. First, they would raise issues as puzzles: "Why did we do this?" or "What is the reason for that?"

Most of the time, no one really knew why things were done the way they were done. It was just "Well, we have always done things that way." So we would discuss ideas about how to do things differently, and the office staff had terrific ideas to make the clinic run better.

It was hard for the doctors, of course, because they were not used to people questioning their authority or ways of doing things. I'm not sure the doctors always appreciated how things changed because, just like at camp, Temperature Reading empowered the staff to say what they think and to raise their concerns. It also fostered an atmosphere that kept the group focused on making things work better. I think even the docs would agree that our service has improved because of the ideas we generate in staff meetings.

A second-year camper and mom said:

After our first year at camp, our son came home and shared with his friends his newfound skill at board games. It was so great to see this group of ten-year-old boys unplugging from electronic toys to play board games together.

Another long-time camper and organizational consultant related:

When I started my leadership-training firm, Virginia reminded me that "all issues are family-of-origin issues." I remember thinking to myself, "Yeah, I know that, and I know it works at camp, but I'm working with business types. No way are they going to let me go in that direction." It was not long before I knew that if I wanted to help people improve their leadership skills, I had to help them understand how their family-of-origin issues affected their skills at work. I decided to follow Virginia's advice and just trust the process. When people identified the problems they were having as leaders, I would ask: "Does any of this feel familiar to you? Did you experience this as a child?" I was amazed that everyone was not only willing to talk about these experiences, but they were open to learning ways to minimize their own reactions.

Some similar things arose for one Committee member and former executive:

> After my first year at camp, I went back to work just full of what I had learned and ideas about how to apply that learning at work. I worked as a manager in a competitive business atmosphere that was a universe away from Family Camp. In the beginning, my staff just put up with my crazy new ideas. First, I used Temperature Reading in team meetings, and that went over okay. Not only did people on my team use it, but they also took it back to the people they supervised and used it with those teams.
>
> I was not as successful when I introduced the Change Model. I don't know if the training itself was the problem or if the ideas were a little too threatening. The ideas never got used the way I hoped. However, when our business was bought out and major changes began to happen, I did hear people talking about the Change Model, so I know they got something from the training.
>
> When the new bosses took over, I tried to help the new manager use Temperature Reading as a tool to improve his meetings. I learned then that unless the leader of the group understands and is committed to the purpose behind the technique, even Temperature Reading will fail. The boss was willing to try the idea, but he wasn't able to listen to the staff. He needed to react, and he was often defensive when people raised their concerns or had ideas about how to do things differently. In the end, it just died of its own weight.
>
> Overall, I think the things I introduced from sfc made a difference. Even though I no longer work there, and there is a totally different management running the place, some of the units still use Temperature Reading. In fact, the one cohesive unit to survive all the changes is the unit that continues to practice those skills.

A long-time camper and retired social worker remembered:

> Each camp, I found something that I took back to my work. The technique that I used the most is the family map. We did this exercise as families at camp. Each family drew a map of the way they see the family now and a map of how they would like the family to be. I adapted this exercise for use by social work supervisors. I had them draw a map of the unit of social workers that they supervise as they are now and a map of how they would like them to be. I was amazed

at how willing these jaded social workers were to do the exercise as well as how much they learned from the experience.

A Committee member and nonprofit agency officer said:

> I use the consensus decision-making model in my work with nonprofit and government organizations. I first used it with our agency's board of directors and, despite their initial hesitancy, they have found the model beneficial.
>
> I also sit on a community board made up of nonprofit agency representatives and representatives of county agencies. These are folks who often disagree on issues and frequently get stuck in their positions. When I suggested that we not vote on issues but rather make our decisions by consensus, some people were uncomfortable. Nevertheless, they were willing to try it and so far, it has worked well. I think it has also led to more understanding between the different groups and less rigid positions.

A long-time camper and schoolteacher reported:

> Temperature Reading is a wonderful tool to use in a classroom. I introduced it my own classroom and then encouraged other teachers to do the same. In one year, all the teachers began to use it in their classrooms. At the end of that year, we had an all-school assembly and planned to show a movie. Of course, the projector broke down and it was going to take at least ten or fifteen minutes to get a replacement. Well, you would expect bedlam to break out, but instead we just had an all-school Temperature Reading. It was amazing. I know Virginia would have been proud!

Expanding the Satir Family Community

sfc members have also been involved in the creation of or planning for other intentional communities. One sfc camper said:

> We started working on developing a family camp in Santa Barbara during the time when sfc was not accepting new campers. We are a family camp that brings together people who share common interests. Most of our program is like sfc's Free University day. Our campers offer groups and activities for the entire camp on a daily basis. We do have a therapeutic component, but it is self-led. We call that component "The Talking Circle." People come together to talk about concerns or interests. Sometimes, we talk about parenting issues; other times, we

may talk about community issues. People come to share and listen. Instead of having a group leader, we use a Talking Stick that we pass from person to person to indicate who wants to speak. Although the Talking Circle is an important part of our camp, our camp is not as focused on the therapy or support groups as sFc.

People come to the camp pretty much the same way that people come to sFc. Existing campers extend an invitation to people they know. We also have a committee that plans the camp, and they decide who will attend the camp. In the beginning, most of the people came from one community and already knew each other, but now we have people who come from all over California as well as from other states.

In contrast to the preceding group, which started as an outgrowth of some campers' sFc experience, another group is planning a Family Camp with closer ties to Virginia and her methods. An sFc camper who works in an academic setting has brought together leading Satir therapists and scholars in her area to replicate a Family Camp based on the Satir model. A founding member of that camp describes other premises they want to include:

We are leaning towards an Experiential Family Therapy orientation and are trying to incorporate The Way of the Council (Native American) and Non-Violent Communication into our methods. We also plan to focus on "sustainable living."

The Satir Intentional Community Model on a World Stage

At the time of Virginia's death, she was developing intentional communities as a way to enhance world peace. She believed that when people connect in communities designed to help them achieve their human potential, they also connect on a spiritual level, which then creates a new universal consciousness and builds world peace (Satir et al., 1991, p. 81). Laura Dodson and others continue Virginia's work on the international level by working with communities in the former Soviet Union, among other countries.

On the world stage, how applicable is the wisdom of Virginia's work? Consider community development on a grand scale, particularly the development of countries as communities. Today, many third-world countries require vast amounts of support to survive, never mind develop. Attempts to help these nations require understanding of how families, then communities, and finally nations develop.

Virginia's ideas can help people understand how these struggling nations can recover after destabilization by a foreign element such as a rebellious or invading force.

Today, for example, Iraq is in the midst of the stage of Rebellion. Initially, right after the initial phase of Operation Iraqi Freedom, energy focused on the Definition and the Establishment stages regarding a new national purpose and structure. The energy of Iraqis focused initially on survival and meeting essential needs. However, as the country rebounded from the war's initial aftermath, the Iraqi government faced its postwar inability to meet everyone's needs fairly and equitably. In this stage, new and unpredictable patterns have emerged and now present unique and unexpected challenges for the people of the country. The same challenges affect all the other nations that have a stake in the outcome and redevelopment of Iraq and its many communities.

Unfortunately, Iraq seems to be fixed in the stage of Rebellion and unable to move on to Redefinition. Attempts to redefine the structure have met with limited degrees of acceptance and much disagreement. As a result, Iraq must return to the initial stage of Definition. This lack of progress is found in many communities that never achieved Synergy or in which the community structures that were synergistic have been destroyed. African nations whose members were forced into slavery and sent to a foreign country and Native American communities whose members were forced from their lands are other examples of nations where all elements of the structure of the developed communities were destroyed. As with Iraq, these communities were forced back to the beginning developmental stages: Definition and Establishment.

In many ways, Satir Family Camp was the beginning of Virginia's drive to achieve world peace by building intentional communities. This book continues that effort by sharing the untold story of Satir Family Camp with a wider audience. It is our hope that the story of sfc will inspire others to create new ways to use Virginia's wisdom to enhance individual, family, and community lives and to follow her path to world peace.

Using Satir Principles to Develop Intentional Communities

Satir principles and methods provide a unique framework for people interested in developing intentional communities. Virginia understood that individuals have an inherent longing to belong. In this day of isolation and electronic social connections, the need to be seen, heard, and supported as an individual grows exponentially. Even as families rush from event to event, they become isolated and lonely in the midst of all their busyness. Where families once turned to their extended family and communities for support and recognition, modern life has replaced human connections with social networks on computers.

The intentional community movement developed as a response to the increasing isolation and disconnection that prevails in our technological society. Many kinds of intentional communities exist. Some share religious beliefs, some form to establish or expand social connections, and others come together because of common interests such as drama, art, or music. The Burning Man Festival, ashrams, Rosie and Kelli O'Donnell's annual cruise for gay and lesbian families, communes in various locations throughout the world, and even summer camps for children are all examples of intentional communities.

Many communities come together for a single week each year; others, for longer. Virginia held annual Process Communities in which people lived together for a month. Some communities, such as the co-housing movement, are for people who wish to live full time in an intentional community.

This book depicts the intentional-community model, which helps describe and understand the stages a community can expect to go through as it begins and then thrives through the years. As discussed in the Definition stage, communities begin by defining their organizational principles. The following statements describe the principles that underlie an intentional community based on Satir principles and philosophy.

- It is a community that brings together families of all kinds to live together for a specified time each year.
- It is defined by and operates on Satir principles and theories.
- It uses Satir methods, including family and group therapy, to foster and maintain connections among community members.
- It practices process and makes decisions via consensus.

Key Elements of a Satir-based Intentional Community

The key elements needed to design and implement a Satir-based intentional community include:

1. Structure
2. Nonhierarchical governance

3. Satir-based therapeutic services
4. Growth-enhancing community activities
5. Supportive physical environment

Structure

A Satir-based intentional community establishes a structure that addresses individual and community concerns in a way that supports rather than divides the community. The structure provides a place and time for the entire community as well as its governing body to meet and plan. At sfc, structure includes the daily community meetings (Temperature Readings), the weeklong community encampment, and the quarterly Committee meetings. The structures allow the community to create and modify how the community works together on a daily, weekly, and yearly basis.

Nonhierarchical Governance

Satir values reflect the principle that all people have value by virtue of being human. Nonhierarchical governance exemplifies that value. It views all individuals as equal and does not define people by status, role, or age. Nonhierarchical government involves all members, including children, in the running of the community. In the Satir model, the daily Temperature Reading assures that all participants, particularly the children, have a voice in the direction of as well as the daily issues that affect the community.

The community as a whole generates and approves governance decisions. Group processing and making decisions by consensus assures that the entire community as well as its governing body adhere to the principle that a Satir community is nonhierarchical and that every voice is heard and given meaning.

Satir-Based Therapeutic Services

Although Virginia taught that therapy is an equal partnership between client and therapist, she did not preach self-help. Virginia viewed the therapist as a guide to help people take in and understand information about themselves and their history. An intentional community based on Satir methods needs to have Satir-trained therapists who participate in a partnership with the community. The therapists help the community learn about and understand Virginia's principles. The therapists use Virginia's methods to help all community members grow to their full human potential. Satir therapeutic experiences not only affect the lives of the people doing the work, they also enrich the community experience by helping people understand and respect why individuals respond as they do.

It is possible to build community connections in many ways. What is unique about a Satir community is the depth of those connections as well as the growth that individuals experience from their experiences living and sharing in the community.

Growth-Enhancing Community Activities

People in a Satir-based intentional community become part of the community by sharing responsibility for running the community. Even the youngest members help the community function. Community jobs and activities provide ways for all people, no matter how reserved, to make connections and become involved as community members.

A Supportive Physical Environment

The location for an intentional community can vary depending on the purpose of the community and the desire of its members. Whether it is located in a wilderness environment or in a more urban area, it is important that community members work together to meet the fundamental needs of the community. Even in SFC's most primitive camp settings, such as Pico Blanco, the organizers provided food and shelter through an arrangement of hired staff and community ownership of tasks.

If you are reading this book to learn about intentional communities, we suggest that you ask yourself the following questions to help decide if creating or joining an intentional community will meet your needs.

1. What is your community? Examine where and how you make connections with others.
2. What are the underlying principles that create or support the connection? Is your community connection related to spiritual beliefs, common interests, children? If you do not have connections now, what are the reasons or purposes that would help you form a community?

3. Can your existing community connections form the basis of an intentional community? Consider the stages of development outlined in this book. In what stage is your community?
4. If you are forming a community, do you have a group that is committed to similar principles and willing to work with you to begin the development?

Conclusion

In this book, we have shared the magic and the realities of Virginia Satir, the wonder that is known as Satir Family Camp, and the great gifts that can be found in an intentional community. We believe that the wisdom and magic that Virginia provided to the Satir Family Camp community can be used in other communities and someday—just as Virginia always intended—on a national and international level. We end our story with Virginia's words on life congruence, which we believe best reflect the hopes and goal of the Satir Family Camp.

Peace Within, Peace Between, Peace Among

Bibliography

Avanta Network (2007).Website: www.avanta.net

Bonar, R. (2004). E-mail correspondence with authors.

Brothers, B. J. (1983). Virginia Satir: Past to present. *Voices: The Art and Science of Psychotherapy, 18* (Win): 48–56.

———. (1998). Virginia Satir, in M. Suhd et al., *Virginia Satir: Her life and circle of influence.* Palo Alto, CA: Science and Behavior Books.

Crane, L. (1999). *Reflections on Satir Family Camp 1999,* Masters thesis, Regis University School of Professional Studies.

Esalen (2002). Website: www.itp-life.com/esalen

Institute for International Connections for Personal and Cultural Growth (IIC), 2007. Website: www.peoplemaking.org

Isles, R. (2002). E-mail correspondence with authors.

Loeschen, S. (1991). *The secrets of Satir: Collected sayings of Virginia Satir.* Palm Springs, CA: Event Horizon Press.

Millman, D. (1995). *The laws of spirit: A tale of transformation.* Tiburon, CA: H. J. Kramer.

Nerin, W. (1986). *Family reconstruction: Long day's journey into light.* New York, W.W. Norton & Co.

Satir Family Camp Committee (1980–2004). Minutes of quarterly Committee meetings. Ventura, CA: Satir Family Camp, Inc.

Satir Family Camp Mission Statement. Ventura, CA: Satir Family Camp, Inc.

Satir Family Camp Handbook (1984, 1996, 2005). Ventura, CA: Satir Family Camp, Inc.

Satir, V. and Baldwin, M. (1983). *Satir step by step: A guide to creating change in families.* Palo Alto, CA: Science & Behavior Books.

Satir, V. and Banmen, J. (1984). *Virginia Satir verbatim.* SeaTac, WA: Avanta Network.

Satir, V.; Banmen, J.; Gerber, J.; Gomori, M. (1991). *The Satir model family therapy and beyond.* Palo Alto, CA: Science and Behavior Books.

Satir, V. Archives (1916–93) Santa Barbara, CA: Special Collection, Davison Library, University of California.

Satir, V. (1964). *Conjoint family therapy A guide to theory and technique.* Palo Alto, CA.: Science and Behavior Books.

Satir, V. (1972). *Peoplemaking.* Palo Alto, CA: Science and Behavior Books.

Satir, V. (1986). *The teachings of Virginia Satir, Series 1* (5 audiotape lectures by Virginia Satir). SeaTac, WA: Avanta Network.

Satir, V. (1986). *Temperature reading* (videotape). SeaTac, WA: Avanta Network.

Satir, V. (1986). *The process of change* (videotape). SeaTac, WA: Avanta Network.

Satir, V. (1986). *The origins and transformation of survival copings* (videotape). SeaTac, WA: Avanta Network.

Schwab, J. (1990). *A resource handbook for Satir concepts.* Palo Alto, CA: Science and Behavior Books.

Schwartz, J. (2006). Personal interview.

Spitzer, R. (2006). Personal interview.

Suarez, M. (1998). "My connection with *Virginia,*" in M. Suhd et al., *Virginia Satir: Her life and circle of influence.* Palo Alto, CA: Science and Behavior Books.

Suhd, M.; Dodson, L.; Gomori, M. (Eds) (2000). *Virginia Satir: Her life and circle of influence.* Palo Alto, CA: Science and Behavior Books.

Wagner, J. (1987). *The effects of Satir Family Camp on individuals and their families: A qualitative study.* Master's thesis. Encino, CA: California Family Study Center.

Wiglesworth, M. (1991). Papers. Santa Barbara, CA: Virginia Satir Archives, Special Collection, Davison Library, University of California.

Wild, S. (2004). Personal interview.